A Comprehensive Guide to the AFP
Cases in Medicine and Surgery

A Comprehensive Guide to the AFP

Cases in Medicine and Surgery

Dalia Abdulhussein • Alice Lee
Mohammad Fallaha

Imperial College London, UK

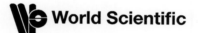
World Scientific

NEW JERSEY · LONDON · SINGAPORE · BEIJING · SHANGHAI · HONG KONG · TAIPEI · CHENNAI · TOKYO

Published by

World Scientific Publishing Co. Pte. Ltd.

5 Toh Tuck Link, Singapore 596224

USA office: 27 Warren Street, Suite 401-402, Hackensack, NJ 07601

UK office: 57 Shelton Street, Covent Garden, London WC2H 9HE

British Library Cataloguing-in-Publication Data
A catalogue record for this book is available from the British Library.

A COMPREHENSIVE GUIDE TO THE AFP
Cases in Medicine and Surgery

ISBN 978-981-123-180-3 (hardcover)
ISBN 978-981-123-306-7 (paperback)
ISBN 978-981-123-181-0 (ebook for institutions)
ISBN 978-981-123-182-7 (ebook for individuals)

For any available supplementary material, please visit
https://www.worldscientific.com/worldscibooks/10.1142/12149#t=suppl

Printed in Singapore

Senior Reviewers

Mr Daniel Leff MBBS BSc FRCS PhD
Consultant in Oncoplastic Breast Surgery and Reader in Breast Surgery at Imperial College London

Mr Sheraz Markar MBBChir, MA (cantab), MRCS (Eng), MSc, PhD
NIHR Clinical Lecturer in General Surgery at Imperial College London

Contents

Preface

We are three surgical academic foundation trainee doctors working in one of the most competitive, academic foundation programme posts in London. We all managed to secure our first-choice job, and this is largely due to attaining a good score at the interview, which for most deaneries makes up the majority of your score. Careful preparation for the interview is therefore vital. We have provided you with a comprehensive guide of how to approach the different types of interviews you may encounter, based on our own experiences. We hope that you will find this guide useful and we wish you all the success in your application process.

Dalia, Alice and Mo

Introduction

1.1 What is the AFP?

The Academic Foundation Programme (AFP) is a 2-year programme of training that takes place in the first two years following graduation from medical school. It can be used as a replacement for the 2-year foundation programme that all medical school graduates apply for in their final year at university.

The conventional Foundation Programme (FP) consists of six 4-month-long placements that run over the course of two years, rotating through a mixture of medical, surgical and community placements. At the end of these two years, doctors are able to apply to any of a variety of training pathways, including GP training, surgical training, medical training or the academic clinical fellowship, amongst others. The point of this 2-year training pathway is to take doctors who have recently qualified, and train them to be fully qualified and licensed to practice independently.

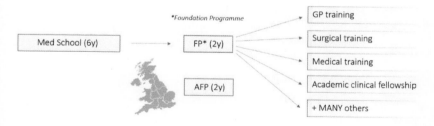

By comparison, the AFP consists of five 4-month-long placements, once again consisting of a mixture of surgical, medical and community placements, in addition to a 4-month-long academic block. The exact nature of this academic block will depend on which type of AFP a candidate opts for, but candidates can choose topics that appeal to them when applying (see Section 1.2 [*What Can I Do My AFP in?*]).

The AFP therefore contains all of the goodies associated with its FP counterpart, namely, time spent on the ward, on calls, nights, and weekends spent working. At the end of it, doctors are fully licensed to practice and the same training paths available to FP graduates are available to AFP graduates too.

In addition, however, AFP doctors have access to the aforementioned 4-month research block, which acts as a protected time to conduct research activities. In some cases, this block is completely protected and contains no clinical work whatsoever, although many AFP placements continue to keep trainees on the on-call rota during this period.

AFP doctors also have an assigned research supervisor, in addition to the education and clinical supervisors provided to them from the FP. This research supervisor acts as a point of contact to help guide and direct the AFP research project conducted by the trainee, but also to help provide mentorship and career planning support.

There are a whole host of additional resources available to AFP doctors, which may vary from deanery to deanery. Most jobs will include access to courses covering research and teaching skills, often at a heavily subsidised (sometimes completely) price. Other jobs will offer access to evening lectures and regional meetings, offering ample opportunity to network with inspiring colleagues, and present preliminary research findings. Sometimes, deaneries offer additional training and certification to AFP doctors, for example, in the form of additional teaching certificates to enhance the candidate's skill set and portfolio. Financial support, in the form of grants and additional funds, is available with some AFP jobs too.

1.2 What Can I Do My AFP in?

There are a variety of research topics available through AFPs, and most jobs nowadays are "themed" (i.e., when you apply, you know what the type and focus of the research project are). Generally speaking, most AFPs can be separated based on the three different types of content of the research block:

1) Research
2) Medical Education
3) Leadership and Management

There are occasionally AFP jobs that have a research focus not included in the above categories (for example, informatics), but these are uncommon. In most cases, the 4-month block in which the research is conducted — the "academic block" — is during the second year of the 2-year AFP. Many AFP doctors, however, contact their supervisor earlier than their block, often in their first year, to decide on the precise nature of the research project and to perform some preliminary reading prior to commencing the project. Some AFP jobs are advertised with the lead supervisor and one or two proposed titles research titles, with some advertising the specific project and role that a successful applicant will assume. Other jobs are less specific, providing greater flexibility (but also responsibility for securing a project) for the successful applicant. The details of all of these jobs can be found through Oriel.

1.3 Why the AFP?

As mentioned prior, the AFP confers a number of advantages over the conventional FP training route as a result of the additional opportunities on offer to candidates. AFP doctors benefit from protected time in which to conduct research, allowing them to immerse themselves in the subject area more easily than individuals who opt to perform research work alongside full-time clinical commitments. This protected time allows a candidate to develop additional skills in research and provides the opportunity to develop research methods and writing skills, which will prove particularly useful to those who are keen to pursue academic careers.

Teaching courses are often provided by deaneries to AFP candidates, which are sometimes even paid for in their entirety. The AFP also provides access to library resources and journals (an expensive and often overlooked benefit of being affiliated with a university), which is often a prerequisite to performing research.

In addition, the AFP also provides additional mentorship and networking opportunities, providing AFP doctors with additional support, knowledge, and guidance to plan future academic careers. The AFP block also provides some variety from the usual ward-work and on-calls from the foundation programme, allowing doctors to pursue additional academic interests.

There are few drawbacks of the AFP, if any. A consequence of the 4-month academic block is less clinical time compared to FP doctors.

However, this is largely negated by the increasing adoption of academic foundation trainees remaining on the on-call rota during their academic block.

1.4 How Do I Apply for the AFP?

At the time of writing (July 2020), applications for the AFP are done using the same online portal (*Oriel*) used to apply for the FP, and applications are made alongside the FP application. All medical students need to apply for the FP but have the option of applying for the AFP. Applicants can apply to a maximum of two deaneries as part of their AFP application; the deadline for application is usually at the end of the second week of October of the final year.

The precise nature of the application form will vary from deanery to deanery, but usually involves information about personal details, additional degrees, publications, presentations and prizes. Many deaneries use "white space" questions as part of the application process; these will be discussed in detail in due course.

Applications are then ranked, with candidates then shortlisted for interviews using shortlisting criteria, which once again, varies from deanery to deanery. Successfully shortlisted candidates are then invited to interviews, usually held between November and January of the final year of medical school, prior to offers being sent out sometime in January. Each deanery has their own way of scoring applications, and you are advised to check each deanery website for further details on the scoring process.

Many candidates are concerned about not making the "cut-off" that is sometimes applied before candidates are shortlisted (for example, some deaneries impose a centile cut-off when shortlisting applicants). These cut-offs vary year-on-year, and you lose nothing by applying for the AFP; if you are considering applying, just do it.

1.5 White Space Questions

Some deaneries ask that you submit answers to a series of questions that they supply prior to the interview, the answer to each of which is usually being between 150–250 words. Answering these questions is likely to instil a feeling of nostalgia for applicants, as they are reminded of their time spent writing the very personal statement that secured their place at medical school. Questions can be vague and broad, or direct and specific. Examples include:

- Give an example in which you have participated and contributed to a successful team.
- Please outline your future career aspirations, and how the AFP will help you achieve this.
- Why do you want to do the AFP?

The strategy for successfully answering these questions remains largely unchanged from when you wrote your personal statement five or six years ago. Start by asking yourself what deaneries are looking for in a successful AFP applicant: leadership qualities, the ability to make decisions, teamwork, clinical acumen, evidence of extra-curricular roles, forward-thinking and career planning.

Then, write out all of your achievements during your medical school in a single list. The next step is to tag your experiences with the qualities that they represent and helped you develop, which are the very qualities deaneries are looking for in applicants.

Finally, answer the white space questions using examples of experiences you have undertaken, with each experience used to highlight a different skill or attribute about yourself. It is always a good idea to make a bullet point skeleton plan of the answers to these questions, before embarking on a mission to convert your ideas into prose — this often provides your writing with greater structure and clearer direction.

The act of "trimming the fact" will force you to decide what is relevant and what is not, and in doing so, you will end up with a leaner piece of writing. Make sure that you send your answers to colleagues and supervisors for feedback but remember that too much feedback can become conflicting and difficult to accommodate. Finally, remember that you have a life and/or degree to be working on outside of the white space questions. Many students make the mistake of spending far too much time on these questions — little and often is all that is required.

Key Points	• Not all deaneries require white space questions
	• Keep an up to date list of all your achievements
	• Tag your experiences
	• Overwrite, and then cut

1.6 How Can I Prepare?

Broadly speaking, there are two groups of actions that can be performed to increase the likelihood of being successful when applying for the AFP. These are:

1) Factors that you can change prior to the process
2) Things to make you shine during the process

1.6.1 *Factors that you can change prior to the process*

These are the factors that will influence your pre-interview score and are used in the shortlisting process and outlined in the subsections below. Note that not all deaneries release information.

Factor	Tips
Decile ranking	• Don't dwell on this too much. • Focus on what you can actually change. • Ask your medical school how it uses the components of various years to contribute towards the decile ranking. • Not all deaneries use decile ranking as a cut-off.
Extra degrees	• Again, this is not an area that you should dwell on. • It probably isn't worth doing an extra degree just to score additional points. • If you are doing an extra degree (most commonly as a result of intercalation), note that a higher graduating class usually means more points.
Publications	• Start early. • Starting a project does not necessarily mean you will get a publication. Put in the effort, be consistent, and see the work through to the end. • Seize every opportunity. The more things you take on, the more likely you will publish. • Don't take on more projects than you can handle. You will become overwhelmed, overworked and lose track of the multitude of projects you have started.

Factor	Tips
	• Systematic reviews and audits count too. • Most deaneries will only accept publications that have a PubMed ID (PMID) • Registrars are often just as keen to publish as you are, since publications enhance their applications to further jobs. Ask them for projects.
Presentations	• You should aim to present every publication you get. • Form a research group and work together with like-minded colleagues.
Prizes	• Medical school examination prizes often count, so this part goes hand-in-hand with the points for decile ranking. • Look out for essays.

1.6.2 *Things to make you shine during the process*

Whilst the aforementioned points focused on the elements of your professional development that can be changed months (or even years) before you think about applying for the AFP, the following section pertains to factors that you can change once the application process has begun.

This begins with the **white space questions**, which some deaneries require as part of the AFP application process. These have been covered in the previous section, but many of the concepts covered in Chapter 2 (*The Personal Questions Interview*) will also aid in writing the answers to these questions.

Successful applicants (of which you will be one) will be required to attend an interview. No AFP positions are filled without the candidate being interviewed first. Broadly speaking, there are three types of interviews:

a) The Personal Interview
b) The Clinical Interview
c) The Academic Interview

Not all deaneries use all of these interview types, and some incorporate elements of these interviews as part of multiple mini interviews.

Each of the individual interview types will require a different preparation method, and you may find that you are naturally stronger at one type than the others. Identifying areas of weakness early on in your preparation is the key to success. Unlike in written examinations, candidates are placed under scrutiny during interviews, and it usually isn't possible to score highly when guessing your way through questions. You need to demonstrate confidence and robust knowledge, and it is therefore important to confront and work on your weaknesses.

Chapter
2

The Personal Questions Interview

2.1 What is the "Personal Interview"?

This is the interview component that focuses on exploring your personal attributes and motivations that make you an ideal candidate for the AFP. Questions may be asked as part of a stand-alone interview distinct from academic and clinical interviews or may be integrated within these other interview types. Note that the skills that will be covered in this section overlap to a great extent with the skills that are applicable to the white space questions.

Candidates often find this section of the interview process particularly daunting. Medical school prepares students to deal with clinical scenarios on a daily basis, and those who are academic-minded will likely have at least some awareness of how to read and interpret research. It does not, however, usually prepare students to be able to talk about themselves.

Despite this relative lack of experience, obtaining success in this component of the interview process is actually relatively straightforward. Successful candidates need to demonstrate only two things; firstly, that they are aware of what attributes theoretically constitute a strong AFP doctor, and secondly, that they have experiences that demonstrate that they possess these attributes.

2.2 What Skills are Desirable?

As covered in Chapter 1, the AFP is essentially a collection of extra-curricular research commitments, which are conducted alongside regular clinical commitments over two years. There are a plethora of skills that would therefore benefit those embarking on an AFP. A limited selection is outlined:

Teamwork	In a conventional FP, doctors rotate through teams every four months. In the AFP, candidates must be able to work within their clinical teams whilst also being part of a wider research team. Remember that most AFP doctors arrange their research project during their F1 year, with many undertaking preliminary work during their first year. Being able to work efficiently and effectively within multiple teams, whilst providing a *meaningful contribution*, is a necessary skill.
Leadership	Whilst F1s are the most junior doctors in the hospital, leadership skills are still required. Remember that effective teachers are able to command the attention of their students, and effective leadership often requires demonstration of the other skills listed in this section.
Knowledge	This is a broad term, encompassing clinical knowledge as well as knowledge about research and academic pathways in medicine. Academic foundation doctors have less clinical time than their FP colleagues and are still required to meet the same clinical competencies as non-academic foundation trainees. AFP applicants must therefore enter the start of F1 with excellent baseline clinical knowledge in order to achieve the same competencies in less time, which is why applicants are scored, during the clinical interview, as if they were an F1.
	Clinical knowledge will be assessed in detail in clinical interviews (see Chapter 3), but interviewers may also ask questions enquiring about the awareness of the academic career pathway in general.

Decision making	As mentioned earlier, you have less time and more commitments during the AFP. Candidates must be able to safely and confidently process scenarios (clinical as well as professional) and make decisions.
Extra-curricular activities	The ability to take on extra-curricular (or extra-vocational) activities demonstrates a number of attributes such as time-management and forward-planning, as well as making you a more well-rounded and interesting individual. It will be reassuring to an interview panel to know that you have previously been able to take on extra work alongside your regular commitments and still managed to succeed.
Forward-thinking	The interview panel will want to know that you have given thought to your future career, and whilst they won't necessarily need you to have decided on a particular specialty, they will want to know how your proposed AFP will fit into your longer-term career ambitions.
Communication skills	The interview panel will want to know that you can communicate confidently and succinctly with colleagues so that you can disseminate information efficiently. They will also want to know that you have effective non-verbal communication skills, which will be assessed during the interview. Finally, they will want to know that you have previous writing experience since you will eventually need to write up and disseminate your research.

There are, of course, many other desirable attributes that have not been listed here, and you may come up with some more of your own that may be more relevant to yourself. Some deaneries publish "person specifications" that may list some of the attributes that they feel are found in desirable applicants, and these may form a part of the scoring criteria.

2.3 How Can I Answer Personal Interview Questions?

It is important to note that successful answers will demonstrate awareness about the ideal attributes whilst also showing self-reflection, highlighting how previous experiences demonstrate the development of these abilities. In their own experiences, the present authors have developed and would recommend the use of the **4 Step Model** (see figure below).

The 4 Step Model

1   Pick an experience

2   Pick an ideal attribute

3   Explain how this attribute was developed by this experience

4   State how this will help you in the AFP

Remember that at the interview, panellists will have only a limited amount of time to assess your character, and this will depend largely on how much relevant information about yourself that you are able to deliver to them, whilst simultaneously answering their questions. The 4 Step Model can be applied to personal questions to enable you to speak about yourself and your prior experiences, whilst also making the interview panellists aware that you have the skills required to undertake an AFP.

Note that the model does not need to be applied rigidly; using the same steps in the same order to answer all questions is likely to come across as robotic and artificial. Instead, the order of the steps can be varied, and the amount of time you spend talking about each step will likely vary depending on the exact experience you're referencing.

Before you can apply this model, you'll likely need to remind yourself of all of your experiences and personal attributes. One of the ways in which this can be done is by listing and then tagging them with the skills and attributes that you feel are highlighted by that experience. This technique is covered in Section 1.5 is "White Space Answers".

Ideal attributes are not confined to those listed in the preceding section, so feel free to highlight the ones you feel you possess most strongly. Finally, remember to finish your answer by addressing the point raised by the initial question, and tie up your answer to a logical conclusion.

2.4 How Should I Go About Preparing?

As mentioned earlier, you will only be able to answer questions about your personal attributes, professional experiences and career aspirations if you have taken some time to list and reflect on previous experiences. Make sure you familiarise yourself with this list of experiences and are confident you can talk about each experience, including a description of the experience as well as what you learnt.

Once you have refreshed your memory about your previous experiences and achievements, you should begin to practice answering these questions. Some candidates will find it useful to make notes for the answers to example questions, but you must ensure your answers come across as natural and not overly scripted. Bullet point lists for model answers usually suffice.

The most useful form of preparation for this interview is to actually practice answering the questions. Ideally, you should find someone who is also applying for the AFP and schedule regular practice with him or her to answer questions and give feedback to each other. Commencing preparation six weeks prior to interviews is usually adequate time to receive feedback and improve on your answers.

Key Points	• Be aware of desirable attributes for AFP applicants
	• Reflect on your own experiences and link them to these attributes
	• Utilise the 4 Step Model to structure your answers
	• Give yourself adequate time to practice with someone else (>6 weeks)

2.5 Example Questions

The table below outlines some of the questions commonly encountered during the personal interview.

Category	Questions
General	<ul><li>Tell us about yourself.</li><li>Explain why you believe you should receive this AFP.</li><li>Is it more important to be a good academic, or a good clinician?</li><li>What are your weaknesses?</li><li>Is there a particular aspect of the AFP that you think you would struggle in?</li></ul>
Desirable skills	<ul><li>Give us an example where you have had to demonstrate leadership skills.</li><li>Give us an example of where you have demonstrated exemplary teamwork.</li><li>Tell us about a time where you demonstrated good communication skills.</li></ul>
Research	<ul><li>Outline one research experience you have learnt something from.</li><li>Tell us about your previous research.</li><li>What areas of research are you interested in?</li><li>Tell us about your research skills.</li><li>Have you previously presented research before, and if so, summarise your key findings.</li></ul>
Motivations	<ul><li>Why have you applied for an AFP?</li><li>Why are you interested in research?</li><li>Why have you applied to this particular deanery?</li><li>Why have you applied for an AFP in this particular topic?</li></ul>
Career-planning	<ul><li>How does the AFP fit into your long-term career aspirations?</li><li>What do you see yourself doing in ten years?</li><li>Are you aware of academic career pathways after the AFP?</li><li>Are you planning on undertaking a PhD?</li><li>Which specialty are you most interested in and why?</li><li>Is research something you are looking to continue long term?</li></ul>

Category	Questions
Organisational	• Give us an example of how you have managed your time well.
Extra-curricular	• Tell us about some of your hobbies outside of medicine. • What additional extra-curricular activities did you take part in during medical school?

Worked Examples

Question	Answer
Q. Tell us about yourself	I am a hard-working student with a passion for acute medicine, and I'm always keen to take on additional challenges and roles that will help me develop as an individual. During medical school, I was the events organiser for the Society of Research and Innovation, a role that required me to research and organise a number of evening lectures delivered by external speakers, alongside my regular medical school studies. I found that this role benefitted me in a couple ways; firstly, I learnt a lot about the various academic careers available within medicine, and secondly, I was able to work on my communication skills as I had to secure speakers for these lectures. Learning about this variety of pathways available in clinical academia made me realise the impact clinical academics can have on patients immediately through their clinical work, as well as more generally through their research.

Feedback

This is intentionally quite a broad question and is sometimes used to open up interviews. Stronger candidates will be able to direct their answer to cover their strengths whilst implementing examples to validate their statements. Note that in this particular question, they are asking you to state some attributes about yourself, so step 2 of the 4 Step Model was used first, followed by step 1.

Note also that this answer has deliberately been vague about the "academic careers" in medicine, with the hope of generating a follow-up question from the interview panel (which, of course, the candidate will have anticipated and prepared an answer for).

On a similar note, this candidate has hinted at their future career aspirations (acute medicine), which once again provides an interesting line of questioning for the interviewer.

Q. Tell us about your previous research	I have been fortunate enough to have been part of a couple of research projects. In my third year of undergraduate medicine, I took part in a retrospective cohort study comparing HbA1c levels in patients on metformin and linagliptin. Taking part in this research introduced me to the principles of writing a project proposal and applying for ethical approval for research work, as well as giving me a greater understanding of the research process as a whole, from project conception to manuscript writing. I believe that this holistic understanding of the research process will make it far easier for me to fit into a project during the research component of the AFP job.

Feedback

This candidate has clearly solid research experience under his or her belt but has not been arrogant about his/her achievements. This person demonstrates a holistic understanding of the research process as a whole, and supervisors will appreciate this understanding since a large portion of the time required to conduct research is taken up by grant applications, the writing of project proposals, and obtaining ethical approval. Awareness of the entire research process makes an AFP candidate a very useful member of the team.

Note that the final sentence in this candidate's answer links the answer back to why he or she would be a good candidate for the AFP (step 4 of the 4 Step Model).

| Q. Are you aware of the research career pathways available after the AFP? | Part of the reason why I have applied to the AFP is that I wanted to get exposure and experience in academic medicine prior to pursuing further academic careers. Research is something I have enjoyed doing at medical school, and I have developed a particular interest in population-based research, having done a BSc in Population Health. During my research project for this intercalation, I was able to write and submit the results to an international journal and present the work internationally.

I aspire to undertake an Academic Clinical Fellowship following the AFP, and I hope that the AFP will help me develop the skills required, such as grant applications and higher population-based statistical analysis, to conduct further research in the field of population health. |

Feedback

This candidate has been honest and realistic, by stating that he or she would like to use the AFP to gain experience in clinical academia, before bringing up the fact that he or she was aware that an Academic Clinical Fellowship (ACF) is something that can be performed later down the line, as part of the academic medicine pathway.

Note that the candidate has brought up something that will be interesting to the interviewers (the previous BSc), which will no doubt generate further questions. The candidate has also brought in future career aspirations, which is something that the interviewers did not ask for but is still related to the answer offered by the candidate.

For further information on academic medicine pathways, see the Medical Schools Council website: https://www.medschools.ac.uk/studying-medicine/after-medical-school/academic-medicine

Key Points

- Keep your answers well-structured so that they are easy to follow

- Direct the line of questioning by adding in snippets of information that you know will generate interest and questions from your interviewers

- Be honest

- Approach this interview as if it were a conversation rather than an interview

- Don't be afraid to bring in additional positive attributes about yourself when answering questions, as long as there is relevance

Chapter 3 The Clinical Interview

The clinical component of the interview aims to gain an insight as to whether you would be a **safe** doctor. The focus is on your thought process and approach to the scenario(s). Most often, you will be provided with either a clinical scenario to work through where you will be given investigations and results depending on whether you have asked for them OR you will be given at least three clinical vignettes and you must discuss your approach within the time with limited or no input of the investigations/results from the interviewers.

The best resource to use for this section of the interview is the *Oxford Handbook of Clinical Medicine*, with particular attention to the final chapter, which provides useful flow-diagram summaries on approaches to common clinical emergencies.

3.1 The Generic Approach to the Clinical Interview

3.1.1 *Working through a series of clinical vignettes*

Often, it is important to ensure that you demonstrate to the interviewer that you are a safe clinician. It is always important that an unwell patient's welfare comes before any professionalism issues you may be provided with, for example, assisting a consultant in theatre, dealing with a complaint or providing collateral for the police.

Most often, you will be provided with a very brief history of the patient along with some of their observations. Based on this, you will need to decide who requires clinical attention.

We suggest following the structure below to start your answer to the clinical vignettes.

Structure	Example of Phrasing
1. **Emphasise that safety of patients is a priority**	"Safety of patients is the main priority, therefore, I would prioritise patients who are most unwell…"
2. **Make seniors aware if there is more than one unwell patient**	"I would make my senior (SHO) aware of the other unwell patient and advise the nurse to closely monitor the patient's observations, and to escalate if there is any deterioration."
3. **Get the nurses to carry out investigations on the other patients in the meantime, if necessary**	"I would like to tell the nurses to get an ECG trace/take blood/site a cannula/regular observation on the other two patients in the meantime."
4. **State the most worrying concerns for each of the patients with a brief list of differentials**	"With this patient I am most worried about…" "Differentials would include…"
5. **Carry out the A to E assessment for the first patient**	"I would follow the ALS approach and carry out a systematic primary survey using the A to E assessment…"
6. **Suggest a definitive management plan (includes alerting the appropriate senior)**	"After assessing the patient, I would like to handover for a senior review/refer to…"
7. **Briefly discuss management of the remaining patients**	"For this patient the main clinical issue is… therefore, I would like to obtain the following investigation…. management options include the following…"

Often this structure can be memorised using the acronym "**RATE**":

R — recognise the main issue
A — assess the patient using A to E approach
T — treat the main issue
E — escalate to seniors as appropriate

3.1.2 *Working through a long clinical case*

Often, in long-case discussions, the examiner will pose questions throughout the encounter and will give information guided by your responses. The key questions to think about when being presented with a case are:

1.   What are the main clinical issues in this case? Which of them are life threatening?
2.   What are the differential diagnoses?
3.   What are the main points to focus on during the assessment of this patient?
4.   What is the definitive management?

3.2 The A to E Management of an Acutely Unwell Patient

Being aware of the ALS approach and carrying out a primary survey using the A to E approach is key to the clinical interview. You will only need to talk through this approach for one of the clinical scenarios.

"I would follow the ALS approach and carry out a systematic primary survey using the A to E assessment..."

AIRWAY	
Assessment	Intervention
1. If the patient is vocalising, then I would assume that the airway is patent. 2. If they are not verbally responsive, I would assess the	1. Immobilise the C-spine if not cleared. 2. Deliver 15L O_2 via Non-rebreathe mask. 3. Airway manoeuvres: head tilt and chin lift (jaw thrust if C-spine injury).

AIRWAY	
Assessment	**Intervention**

airway using a **Look, Listen, Feel** approach:
a. **Look:** for any foreign body/ airway secretions that can be suctioned.
b. **Listen:** for upper airway sounds that may indicate obstruction such as stridor, gurgling.
c. **Feel:** for expired air.
	4. Airway adjuncts: Guedel/ oropharyngeal or nasopharyngeal airways.
	5. If airway patency is still not achieved, put out a peri-arrest call.
	  a. Definitive treatment will be an endotracheal intubation.
	  b. **NB:** If not breathing + no pulse → commence CPR.

BREATHING	
Assessment	**Intervention**

1. I would like to check the patient's respiratory rate and saturation.
2. Assess the efficacy of breathing using a **Look, Listen, Feel** approach.
  a. **Look:** use of accessory muscles, chest expansion
  b. **Listen:** vesicular BS? Any added sounds?
  c. **Feel:** tracheal deviation and chest expansion
	1. Sit the patient up
	2. Bedside tests:
	  a. Arterial Blood Gas if sats <94% on air
	3. Imaging:
	  a. (Portable) chest X-ray
	4. Titrate oxygen according to needs
	  a. Normally aim for 94–98%
	  b. If chronic CO_2 (COPD patients), retainers aim for 88–92%
	5. Investigate and treat the cause
	  a. Infection → Antibiotics
	  b. Pulmonary Oedema → Diuretics
	  c. Pulmonary embolus → Anticoagulation

CIRCULATION	
Assessment	**Intervention**

1. Check the patient's Heart Rate, Blood Pressure, Temperature and Urine Output
2. Examine the patient's:
  a. **Pulse:** rate, rhythm, volume and character
  b. **Heart sounds**
  c. **Capillary refill time (central)**
	1. Initially I would:
	  a. Take blood tests for FBC/ UE/CRP...
	  b. Site a cannula
	  c. 12-Lead ECG to look for any dynamic changes...
	  d. Catheter for accurate UO
	  e. If necessary, start on cardiac monitoring
	2. If the patient is haemodynamically unstable:
	  a. Give a fluid challenge to see if they respond: STAT 500 ml bolus of normal saline (250 ml if fluid overloaded/elderly)
	  b. Re-assess BP and give further fluid challenge
	  c. If no improvement after two fluid boluses, escalate

DISABILITY	
Assessment	**Intervention**
1. I would assess the patient's **Glasgow Coma Score** 2. I would check the patient's **pupils** (equal and reactive to light/accommodation) 3. I would like to know the patient's **BMs** 4. I would perform a brief **neurological examination** assessing the tone/power/ reflexes in the four limbs	1. GCS <8 indicates an AIRWAY problem (equivalent to an AVPU of P, i.e., responsive to pain only) 2. Intervention as appropriate according to cause

EXPOSURE	
Assessment	**Intervention**

1. I would fully **expose the patient** and look for any skin changes, bleeding or hidden injuries
2. If appropriate I would perform:
  a. An abdominal examination +/− PR exam
  b. Examine the calves to assess for infection/fluid status/thrombus
	Escalate as appropriate and treat the cause
	
	1. Activate Major Haemorrhage Protocol (when SBP <90 and there is evidence of bleeding)

Key Points
- Remember that the most clinically urgent problems are **AIRWAY** problems, followed by **BREATHING** problems, followed by **CIRCULATION**, followed by **DISABILITY**.
  - That is to say that a breathing problem will kill you before a circulation problem.
  - So, a pulmonary embolus will kill you before a major haemorrhage.
- Never move onto the next assessment if there is an issue with the current.
  - For example, if a patient is saturating at 76% on air, it is more appropriate to fix this, re-assess, and when you have solved the issue to move on to C.

- Note that it may be appropriate to outline briefly the assessment of each of the components but to focus on the assessment most appropriate to the clinical scenario in question.
  - So, if a patient's BP is 88/54 and the rest of the observations are fine, then it is not entirely appropriate to talk through the whole airway algorithm. Instead, just mention that airway is patent as the patient is verbalising, and then move on to the next stage.

3.3 Medical Ethics and Law: Core Components Useful for the Interview

Being aware of some of the key ethical principles is important for the interview, as there may be scenarios where you will need to draw on this knowledge. These principles are also useful for the academic interview.

The Four Ethical Principles	
Autonomy (and confidentiality)	Patients have the right to make decisions regarding their own care
Beneficence	Clinicians must act in the best interests of their patients
Non-maleficence	Clinicians must do no harm
Justice	Fair and equal treatment of patients irrespective of background

Remember that hospital admissions can be either:

- **Voluntary**, i.e., a patient is sick, and they bring themselves in.
- **Under the Mental Health Act 2007**
  - This is the compulsory admission and treatment of mental illness patients who are considered at risk of themselves/others.
  - Section 5(2) is the doctor's holding power for in-patients, i.e., can be used if a patient with acute psychosis and a known background of schizophrenia is attempting to leave the ward.
- **Under the Mental Capacity Act 2005**
  - When you must act in the patient's best interests if they are deemed to lack capacity.
  - A patient has capacity if they are able to:
    a. Understand information
    b. Retain information
    c. Use/weigh up information as part of his or her's decision-making process
    d. Communicate decisions

— For example, if a patient is attempting to leave the ward (he or she is acutely intoxicated to alcohol/have delirium), keeping them in hospital is acting in their best interest as they lack the capacity to make decisions regarding their healthcare. In such instances, where we are keeping a patient in against their will, it is important to involve the family and fill out a DoLS (Deprivation of liberty status) form explaining why it is in their best interest that we do so.

It is also important to be aware of the circumstances under which confidentiality can be breached, as there may be scenarios where a police officer would like to talk to you regarding an admitted patient. You could **breach confidentiality** under the following circumstances:

1. Sharing information with other healthcare professionals
2. Disclosure required by law:
   a. Death
   b. Termination
   c. Notifiable diseases (**NB:** HIV is not a notifiable disease)
3. Assisting the police:
   a. Driver suspected of offences
      o Suspected terrorist identification
      o Use of weapons, children at risk/safeguarding
4. Disclosure in public interest
   a. Prevention/prosecution of serious crime
   b. Protect patient/others from serious harm

Remember that safeguarding does not exclusively relate to children. You may encounter the issue of safeguarding in many other scenarios, including domestic abuse and neglect from carers towards the patient, which results in their admission. Whenever such issues are suspected, the safeguarding team at the hospital is alerted. It is a professional duty to raise concerns about any patient's welfare.

3.4 Important Non-Clinical Issues for the Clinical Interview

Often, the scenarios will include a non-clinical issue, which you will be called about. This may include things such as dealing with complaints and updating family members.

3.4.1 *Dealing with patients who are aggressive*

1. Identify why the patient is aggressive.
   a. Are they delirious? Are they angry/frustrated with the way their care has been delivered?
   b. It may be appropriate to briefly read through their medical notes.
2. Ensure the environment is appropriate for discussion.
3. Verbal de-escalation in the first instance.
4. If the patient is attempting to leave:
   a. If they have capacity, they must sign a form to say that they wish to self-discharge **against** medical advice.
   b. If they lack capacity, a DoLS form needs to be filled as keeping them in hospital is in their best interest.
5. Pharmacological depressants.
   a. If verbal de-escalation has not worked and the patient is becoming more aggressive, using IM Lorazepam/Haloperidol may be indicated.
   b. Alongside this, ensure they have 1:1 nursing.

3.4.2 *Dealing with complaints/an angry relative*

1. Familiarise yourself with the patient's story.
2. What is their relation to the patient? Are they the next of kin?
   a. Remember you can only disclose information at the consent of the patient, and if they lack consent, then this decision would usually reside with the next of kin.
3. Ensure the environment is appropriate for discussion.
4. What is the issue?
   a. Is there anything that can be done about it?
   b. Do not apologise for what has been done so far. This may indicate there has been a mismanagement of the patient, when there may not have been.
5. Point them towards the PALS team (patient advice and liaison team) where formal complaints can be made.

3.5 Common Scenarios and Worked Answers for Examples

As mentioned previously, the best way to prioritise clinical scenarios is based on clinical urgency. In order to decide for this, it is important to be able to recognise some of the most common pathologies and which problem category they mainly come under. Below is a table that outlines the most common pathologies you will encounter in your interview and which system they mostly affect.

Problem	Pathologies
Airway	<ul><li>Any cause of LoC (GCS <8), for example:<ul><li>Seizures: Epileptic, Metabolic (electrolytes, glucose), infections (meningoencephalitis)</li><li>Head Injury</li></ul></li><li>Anaphylaxis</li></ul>
Breathing	<ul><li>Asthma</li><li>COPD</li><li>Pulmonary embolus</li><li>Pulmonary oedema</li><li>Pneumothorax</li></ul>
Circulation	<ul><li>Shock<ul><li>Septic: head/chest/abdomen/urine</li><li>Haemorrhagic: upper GI bleeding, AAA rupture, PR bleeding</li></ul></li><li>Brady/tachy-arrhythmias</li><li>Myocardial infarction</li><li>Aortic dissection</li><li>Cardiac tamponade</li></ul>
Disability	<ul><li>Hyperglycaemia<ul><li>DKA</li><li>HHS</li></ul></li><li>Hypoglycaemia<ul><li>**NB:** Can cause LoC/Seizures</li></ul></li><li>Delirium</li><li>Drug overdoses</li></ul>
Exposure	<ul><li>Hypothermia</li></ul>

Often, candidates have different experiences of the clinical interview, with some being asked no questions and are expected to run through the cases alone throughout the 10-minute period with no additional observations/investigations, while others have more frequent questioning. Below are some examples of clinical cases for you to practice with. We outlined brief approaches to each example.

Short Cases Examples

Short Cases: Example 1

You are the surgical FY1 on-call. During a busy night, you get bleeped about the following in quick succession:

1. A 76-year-old who is D2 post-op for an anterior resection has suddenly desaturated at 88% on air. His RR is 24, BP is 112/70 and HR is 101.
2. A 40-year-old who is admitted with likely gallstone pancreatitis, is in an extreme amount of pain and is starting to distress the other patients. His HR is 112, BP is 150/90, sats 95% on air, RR of 20.
3. A 56-year-old gentleman who has been admitted with loin-to-groin back pain, presumed to be secondary to a renal stone that has become suddenly hypotensive. His HR is 121, BP is 90/58, RR is 16, sats 965 on air.

Your consultant wants you to attend theatre to assist with an emergency appendicectomy in a 10-year-old.

Tell us how you would approach this clinical scenario

1. Emphasise that safety of patients is a priority	The safety of patients is the main priority. Therefore, I would prioritise patients who are the most unwell. In this case, the main issues are:
	1. Breathing problem in patient 1
	2. Uncontrolled pain in patient 2
	3. Circulation problem with patient 3
	4. Consultant needing assistance
	Based on this, I believe patient 1 is the most unwell, followed by patient 3. I would then address patient 2 and ensure I have made my consultant aware that it is a busy shift and that I have more than one unwell patient to attend to. Therefore, I will not be able to join him in the theatre.

2. Make seniors aware if there is more than one unwell patient	Seeing that there are two patients, I am most worried about, I would make my SHO aware of patient 2 and see if he or she can assess him.
3. Get the nurses to carry out investigations on the other patients in the meantime, if necessary	Whilst I go to assess patient 1, I would like to advise the nurses to do the following for patient 3: • Take blood: FBC, UE, CRP, Clotting, Crossmatch • Site a cannula • ECG trace • Monitor urine output • Regular observations and escalate if there is further deterioration

4. State the most worrying concerns for each of the patients with a brief list of differentials	• **Patient 1** has suddenly desaturated. In a post-operative patient, I would be most worried about a Pulmonary Embolus.
	  o Other differentials: post-operative atelectasis, Pneumonia, Pneumothorax.
	• **Patient 3** is haemodynamically unstable and in this context, I would be most worried about a rupture of his AAA.
	  o Other differentials: sepsis, bleeding from elsewhere, tachyarrhythmia.
	• **Patient 2's** observations are stable; his high BP and HR may be secondary to anxiety/pain, which is common in pancreatitis patients.

5. Carry out the A to E assessment for the first patient	I would like to assess **patient 1** first, I would follow the ALS approach and carry out a systematic primary survey using the A to E assessment:

A	• If the patient is verbalising, I would assume the airway is patent.
	• If the patient is not vocalising, then I would assess the airway using a look, feel, listen approach and then attempt simple airway manoeuvres in the first instance, followed by airway adjuncts. If I am still unsuccessful, I would contact an anaesthetist urgently (peri-arrest call).
	I would also put the patient on a 15L non-rebreathe mask.
B	• I would like to know his sats and RR.
	• I would then like to briefly examine him, looking for any signs of infection/pneumothorax using the look, feel, listen approach.
	• I would then like to get an ABG to assess for any respiratory failure.
	• I would then like to obtain a CXR.
	• I would re-check the sats and titrate the oxygen requirement, aiming for sats of 88–92% or 94–98%, if not a chronic retainer.
C	Once I am happy with the patient's breathing, I would like to assess his circulation. Currently, he is haemodynamically stable but has signs of early shock as he is tachycardic. I would like to:
	• Examine him.
	• Send him for blood tests: FBC, UE, CRP, Clotting +/– D-Dimer (based on Well's score), Crossmatch.
	• Ensure he has good IV access.

		• Interpret his ECG. • Monitor UO. • Commence him on cardiac monitoring. • Consider giving a fluid challenge (250 ml in this case if he has a PE, he may have some element of right heart strain).
	D **E**	I would then re-assess A to C and complete my assessment by assessing D and E. D: GCS, BMs, Neurological exam E: assess calves for DVT
6. Suggest a definitive management plan (which includes alerting the appropriate senior)		After assessing the patient, I would like to discuss with my senior if further imaging/treatment may be necessary, seeing as clinical suspicion for a PE is high. 1. Definitive diagnostic investigations include CTPA if his kidney function is good. 2. Definitive management will depend on if he is haemodynamically stable or not. Seeing as he is haemodynamically stable, he would be on a treatment dose LMWH (as per local protocol). 3. For patients who are not haemodynamically stable, thrombolysis may be considered but this is a senior-led decision.
7. Briefly discuss management of the remaining patients		I would take a similar approach to assess **patient 3** with a focus on his circulation. I am most worried about an AAA rupture. I would like to ensure the following has been done prior to escalating to a senior:

- Blood tests: FBC, UE, CRP, Clotting, Crossmatch.
- Ensure he has good IV access.
- Monitor UO (ensure catheter is in).
- Commence him on cardiac monitoring.
- Give him 2×500 ml fluid boluses.
- If there is evidence of an AAA rupture, it would be appropriate to put out a **Major Haemorrhage** call.
- If clinical suspicion for an AAA rupture is high, an emergency laparotomy is indicated as the definitive management.

Next, I would like to assess **patient 2**, although it is likely that he has no adequate analgesia but it is important to rule out other causes of his pain. Some of the key management options in pancreatitis include:

- NBM to rest the pancreas.
- IV Antibiotics if high inflammatory markers.
- IVF/TPN if being kept NBM >3–5 days.
- Adequate analgesia.
- Exclude ARDS, bowel obstruction or SMV thrombus, which are complications and may account for the pain.

Short Cases: Example 2

You are the medical FY1 on ward cover. You have been bleeped about the following patients:

1. A 80-year-old lady, who has been admitted with delirium likely secondary to a UTI, has just had an unwitnessed fall in the ward and the nurses would like you to assess her.

Short Cases: Example 2

2. A 56-year-old gentleman with a background of HTN, T2DM, Hypercholesterolaemia, who is currently medically fit for discharge after being treated for a CAP, has developed central chest pain. His HR is 101, BP is 100/65, sats 98% on air, and RR is 16.
3. The relatives of a 91-year-old would like to talk to you regarding the care of their mother. They would like to put in a complaint, as they are not happy that she has been made "not for resuscitation" without their consent.
4. A 46-year-old lady who has a background of bipolar disorder has harmed herself in the ward and has slit both her wrists and thighs. The nurses would like you to assess her. Her observations are stable.

How would you proceed?

What are the main clinical issues presented here?

Patient 1	D and E problem — In any patient who has had a fall, the main worry would be a head injury resulting in an intra-cranial bleed. — Other issues include a traumatic bony injury, e.g., neck of femur fracture.
Patient 2	C problem — In any patient with a strong cardiovascular background and complaining of central chest pain, myocardial infarction must always be high on the differential list.
Patient 3	Non-clinical issue
Patient 4	E problem — It would be important to ensure that her observations are stable and that she is well otherwise. — Often, slits to the wrist are superficial.

How would you proceed?

Based on the issues outlined above, the most unwell patients take precedence. Therefore patient 2 (C problem) should be seen first, followed by patient 1 (D and E problem), patient 4, and then patient 3.

How would you assess the patients?

I would follow the ALS approach and carry out a systematic primary survey using the A to E assessment. The focus of the assessment and pertinent points for each patient would be as follows:

Patient 1	A: ensure patent B: ensure sats and RR are stable C: check HR, BP and Temp D: • Assess GCS • Check pupils • Measure BMs • Neurological examination to assess for any deficits E: • Examine joints to assess for any injuries • Look to see if any bruising or sites if bleeding
Patient 2	A: ensure patent B: • Aim for sats >94%. Do not give oxygen if not necessary, as per ACS protocol • Examine the patient and exclude pulmonary oedema (which is a complication of an acute MI) C: • Examine • Send blood tests: FBC, UE, CRP, Clotting, **Troponin** • Ensure he has good IV access • ECG to look for any dynamic changes • Commence him on cardiac monitoring • Monitor UO

Patient 3	Non-clinical issue
Patient 4	A: ensure patent B: ensure sats and RR are stable C: check HR, BP and Temp D: GCS, pupils, BMs, brief neurological examination E: • Assess extent of soft tissue injury • Ensure wounds are washed and dressed

How would you manage the patients?

Some important management points would be:

Patient 1	Ensure provisions are in place to prevent further falls. Consider imaging: — X-rays if suspicious of bony injury. — CT head if this meets the criteria according to NICE (for example, if patient is on DOAC). Treat underlying cause of delirium.
Patient 2	The definitive management of MI depends on whether there is an ST elevation on the ECG or not. — In either case you should immediately make the registrar on-call aware and seek advice. — Follow local guidelines on management.

STEMI	NSTEMI
• STAT Aspirin and Clopidogrel 300 mg • GTN SL spray 400 mcg • IV 10 mg Morphine + metoclopramide 10 mg	• STAT Aspirin and Clopidogrel 300 mg • GTN SL spray 400 mcg • IV 10 mg Morphine + metoclopramide 10 mg • Fondaparinux 2.5 mg SC
URGENT PCI within two hours	Non-urgent angiography +/– angioplasty

Patient 3	Explain that DNACPR is usually a medical decision and the family tends to play an advisory role. — CPR is futile. — DNACPR ensures that the patient would not die in an undignified way.
Patient 4	Ensure the patient has 1:1 monitoring. Assess for further risk. Examine belongings to ensure there is no other way of harming oneself. Consider escalating to psychiatry team to arrange a transfer to a psychiatric hospital.

Short Cases: Example 3

You are the medical FY1 on ward cover. You have been bleeped about the following patients:

1. A 57-year-old, who was admitted with poor oral intake and a background of T2DM, chronic pancreatitis and alcohol excess, begins seizing in the ward.
2. A 19-year-old, who was recently admitted with a fever, headache and aggressive behaviour, has become violent and is attempting to leave the ward.
3. The nurses want you to review a 50-year-old lady who has just had an episode of melaena. Her HR is 110, BP is 97/54, sats 98% on air, RR is 16, and Temp is 37.5°C.
4. You are also asked by the nurses to write an urgent transfer letter for a patient in the CCU who is about to go for an angiogram +/− angioplasty at the local tertiary centre.

How would you proceed?

What are the main clinical issues presented here?

Patient 1	A problem — Patients who are seizing are unable to maintain their own airway.

Patient 2	Patient attempting to leave ward.
Patient 3	C problem — This patient has signs of an UGIB (melaena) and is displaying signs of haemodynamic compromise (compensatory tachycardic).
Patient 4	Transfer of a clinically stable patient to a tertiary centre.

How would you proceed?

Based on the issues outlined above, the most unwell patients take precedence. Therefore patient 1 (A problem) should be seen first, followed by patient 3, patient 2, and then patient 4.

How would you assess the patients?

I would follow the ALS approach and carry out a systematic primary survey using the A to E assessment. The focus of the assessment and pertinent points for each patient would be as follows:

Patient 1	Someone should start timing the seizure. If the seizure lasts > 5 minutes, then a peri-arrest call should be put out. Whilst the patient is having a seizure, he or she should be placed into the recovery position. Ensure the crash-trolley is nearby. Ensure that 20% dextrose and Lorazepam are on stand-by. A: put on a 15L non-rebreathe mask B: check sats during the seizure C: • Send off bloods: FBC, UE, CRP, Prolactin (to see if it is a true seizure), Bone profile, Clotting, and send off a VBG (to check the lactate) • Ensure good IV access D: • Measure BMs (hypoglycaemia is a reversible cause)

Patient 2	Ascertain why this person wanted to leave.
	Assess this person's capacity.
	Read through his medical notes to find out the clinical impression and management.
Patient 3	A: ensure patent B: check sats and RR C:
	• Send blood tests: FBC, UE, LFTs, CRP, Clotting, crossmatch, consider getting a VBG (lactate is a good marker of end organ perfusion, VBG can also give a quick result for the Hb) • Ensure good IV access • Fluid challenge with 500 ml bolus
	D: GCS, BMs, gross neurolgical examination E:
	• Abdominal examination: peritonitic? • PR exam
Patient 4	This is the least priority task — make the nurses aware that you are busy with some unwell patients therefore it will take some time to arrange the letter. See if they can get in contact with someone else to write the letter.

How would you manage the patients?

Some important management points would be:

Patient 1	Once the patient has been seizing for 5 minutes, ensure the following:
	1. Peri-arrest call is put out 2. IV lorazepam (2–4 mg) into a large vein, can give another dose after 10 minutes if no resolution 3. If no IV Access: PR Diazepam 10 mg or Buccal Midazolam 10 mg 4. If no resolution, then anaesthetist will need to decide if phenytoin/phenobarbital infusion should be commenced

Patient 2	If the patient has no capacity, then you will need to fill out a DoLS form. Inform the next of kin that you done so. Arrange for security, if needed, to prevent the patient from leaving the hospital.
Patient 3	For an UGIB: 1. After primary survey, alert your senior of your findings 2. Keep patient NBM and request an OGD 3. Correct clotting abnormalities, omit any DOAC/DAPT 4. Blood transfusion if Hb <70
Patient 4	If there is no time to write a transfer letter and this is delaying the patient's treatment, then it may be appropriate to call the team at the hospital receiving the patient and give a brief handover out of courtesy.

Short Cases: Example 4

You are the medical FY1 on ward cover. You have been bleeped about the following patients:

1. A 62-year-old gentleman who was admitted with palpitations is on telemetry. The nurses ask you to review him as his HR is consistently at 140 bpm and he is beginning to feel a little short of breath. His BP is 90/50, RR is 24, sats 94% on air, and Temp is 36.8°C.
2. **A 50-year-old gentleman admitted with an exacerbation of COPD in the ward has spiked a temperature of 38.1°C. His BP is 110/80, HR 109, sats 89% on air. He states he wants to go home because he feels that the doctors are not helping in any way.**
3. The nurses bleep you to review a patient whose temperature has decreased to 34.5°C (from 36.8°C). His BP is 120/80, HR is 6, RR 16, and sats 98% on air.

How would you proceed?

What are the main clinical issues presented here?

Patient 1	C problem
	— This patient is haemodynamically compromised.
	— The likely issue here is a tachyarrhythmia.
Patient 2	C problem
	— This patient is at risk of sepsis (likely source is chest).
Patient 3	E problem
	— Hypothermic patient.
	— There are many causes, remember that cold sepsis (where the patient has a low temperature) could also be the culprit.

How would you proceed?

Based on the issues outlined above, the most unwell patients take precedence. In this scenario, there are two unwell patients. Therefore, I would like to make my senior aware to see if they are able to attend to one whilst I assess the other. If I was alone, I would assess patient 1 (C problem) first, followed by patient 2 (C problem), and then patient 3.

I would also advise nurses on what to do for the remaining patients whilst I assess the first patient.

How would you assess the patients?

I would follow the ALS approach and carry out a systematic primary survey using the A to E assessment. The focus of the assessment and pertinent points for each patient would be as follows:

Patient 1	A: ensure patent
	B: check sats and RR
	C:
	• Examine: check if HD stable
	• Send blood tests: FBC, UE, Bone profile, Mg, TFT, CRP
	• Ensure good IV access
	• ECG

	• Urine output • Ensure patient has on-going cardiac monitoring • Fluid challenge with 500 ml bolus D: GCS, BMs, gross neurolgical examination E: Fully expose
Patient 2	A: ensure patent B: • Titrate oxygen according to requirements (i.e., Venturi 28%) • Examine • Consider CXR • Consider ABG as septic C: • Send blood tests: FBC, UE, CRP, Blood Cultures, Clotting • Ensure good IV access • ECG • Urine output • Ensure on telemetry • Fluid challenge with 500 ml bolus D: GCS, BMs, gross neurolgical examination E: fully expose
Patient 3	A: ensure patent B: check sats and RR • May need to start patient on warm, humidified oxygen • Order a CXR to exclude a source of infection C: • Examine: check if HD stable • Send blood tests: FBC, UE, Clotting (at risk of DIC), TFT, CRP • Ensure good IV access • ECG (J waves, AF, prolonged QRS)

- Urine output
- Put on cardiac monitoring (at risk of arrest)
- Commence on slow warm IV fluids

D: GCS, BMs, gross neurolgical examination
E: fully expose patient

How would you manage the patients?

Some important management points would be:

Patient 1	Manage as per the Resus Council Tachyarrhythmia algorithm. Management would depend on the presence of adverse signs (SSMH): — Syncope — Shock — Heart Failure — Myocardial Ischaemia Will need to correct any underlying electrolyte abnormalities/causes.
Patient 2	For patients with infective exacerbation of COPD: 1. Bronchodilators: ipratropium bromine 500 mcg and salbutamol 500 mg nebulised 2. Prednisolone 30 mg for 5–7 days 3. IV Antibiotics as per local guidelines Explain to the patient why he is in hospital, clarify any uncertainties and answer questions. Most of the time, patients try to leave the ward due to misunderstandings. Therefore, communication is key.
Patient 3	1. Alert your senior 2. Commence patient on a bear hugger in the first instance 3. If this has not worked, then you may need to re-escalate for consideration of warmed fluid lavage, dialysis or ECMO

Short Cases: Example 5

You are the FY1 on a surgical night shift. You are bleeped by the nurses for the following patients:

1. A 85-year-old gentleman who is day 7 post-anterior resection with loop ileostomy and a background of COPD, HTN and dementia. The nurse has bleeped you as he has just spiked a temperature at 38.0°C. His HR is 114, BP is 90/54, sats 94% on air, and RR is 19. He is complaining of abdominal pain.
2. A 14-year-old boy who is currently six hours nil-by-mouth prior to his appendicectomy and has not had any IV fluids prescribed.
3. A 52-year-old woman, admitted with PR bleeding on a background of haemorrhoids, has become acutely confused and is insisting on being discharged. The nurses want you to review her and prescribe a sedative.

The family of patient 1 has arrived and is requesting an update on his progress and plans for his care.

How would you proceed?

What are the main clinical issues presented here?

Patient 1	C problem — This patient is septic post-operatively.
Patient 2	Stable patient requiring fluids as he is NBM.
Patient 3	D problem — Confused patient who would like to leave.

How would you proceed?

In this scenario, patient 1 should be prioritised, as he is haemodynamically compromised and most likely secondary to sepsis (likely intra-abdominal source). Next, I would like to assess patient 3 as she is attempting to leave and has become confused. Finally, patient 2 needs to be prescribed fluids, as he is NBM.

Whilst assessing patient 1, I would ask the nurses to calm patient 3 and ascertain if she has capacity or not. I would also like them to keep a close eye on patient 2 and ensure his observations are stable and that he is not distressed.

How would you assess the patients?

I would follow the ALS approach and carry out a systematic primary survey using the A to E assessment. The focus of the assessment and pertinent points for each patient would be as follows:

Patient 1	A: ensure patent B: check sats and RR • Consider CXR as part of septic screen • ABG as patient is septic C: • Send blood tests: FBC, UE, CRP, Blood cultures • Ensure good IV access • ECG • Urine output (send off urine cultures) • Ensure has on-going cardiac monitoring • Fluid challenge with 250 ml bolus D: GCS, BMs, gross neurolgical examination E: • Examine abdomen: peritonitic? • In a post-op patient, always consider the risk of anastomotic leak/ abdominal collection
Patient 2	Ensure observations are stable. Briefly assess if the patient is experiencing any symptoms.
Patient 3	Assess if the patient has capacity. Is this a new-onset confusion? If so, then perform an A to E assessment to identify the cause.

How would you manage the patients?

Some important management points would be:

Patient 1	Sepsis 6 management (ensure the following are done during the A to E assessment): • 3 out: urine output, blood cultures, lactate (ABG/VBG) • 3 in: fluids, antibiotics (according to local guidelines), oxygen **qSOFA** is a screening tool which indicated poor outcomes (and therefore need for escalation): 1. Altered mental status (GCS <15) 2. RR >22 3. SBP <100 mmHg
Patient 2	Prescribe fluids as per paediatric maintenance fluid requirements (according to weight): • <10 Kg: 100 ml/kg per day • 10–20 Kg: 1000 mL + 50 ml/kg per day • >20 Kg: 1500 mL + 20 ml/kg per day
Patient 3	If delirious, then treat the underlying cause. If no capacity → DoLS Ensure patient has 1:1 nursing/security to prevent her from leaving.

Long Cases Examples

Long Cases: Example 1

You are the FY1 on take. You have been asked to go and clerk a 21-year-old who has presented with a 4-day history of abdominal pain and vomiting. She is currently in A&E Resus. Her observations are: HR 122, BP 100/72, RR 30, sats 100% on air, and Temp 37.8°C.

What are the most pertinent clinical conditions to consider in this case?

Given this patient's age:

1. Surgical cause of an acute abdomen
   a. Acute appendicitis
   b. Gynaecological pathology
2. Medical causes of an acute abdomen
   a. Infection: gastroenteritis
   b. Inflammation: Inflammatory bowel disease
   c. Metabolic: Diabetic Ketoacidosis

How would you assess this patient?

I would follow the ALS approach and carry out a systematic primary survey using the A to E assessment.

A	If the patient is verbalising, I would assume that the airway is patent.
	I would like to put the patient on a 15L non-rebreathe mask.
B	I would like to check the sats and RR at this point.
	I would like to examine the patient to look for any signs of respiratory distress and auscultate lung fields to exclude infection.
	I would like to request a CXR when the patient is more stable.
C	I would like to examine the patient to see if she is haemodynamically compromised.
	Next, I would like to ensure the patient has good IV access and send blood for the following: FBC, UE, CRP, Clotting, Blood Cultures.
	I would like to obtain an ECG trace.
	I would like to ensure a catheter is inserted for accurate urine output measurement.
	I would also like to ensure that she is on regular telemetry monitoring.
	Finally, I would like to give her a 500 ml fluid bolus and see if her BP responds to this, I would like to repeat this two times, and if her BP remains low, escalate to a senior immediately.
D	I would like to assess her GCS, Pupils and do a gross neurological examination.

> **E** I would like to fully expose as appropriate and examine the following:
>
> - Calves to exclude a DVT
> - Abdomen to exclude an acute abdomen

You are provided with this patient's VBG:

pH 7.299
pCO_2 5.40
pO_2 6.81
HCO_3 15.4
BE −5
Glu 29.1
Lactate 3.4

Is there any other particular investigation you would like which would aid diagnosis?

Blood ketones.

What would be the definitive management?

The most likely diagnosis here is diabetic ketoacidosis, which requires the following criteria to be met:

1. Acidaemia: pH <7.3 or HCO_3 <15
2. Hyperglycaemia: blood glucose >11
3. Ketoneamia: ≥3

The definitive management is usually outlined in hospital guidelines. This includes:

1. Commencing the patient on a fixed rate insulin infusion in order to bring the blood ketones down
   a. If the patient is on long-acting insulin this should be continued.
2. Aggressive fluid resuscitation
3. Hourly VBGs
4. Thrombophylaxis
5. Identification of a trigger and treating the underlying cause

Long Cases: Example 2

You are the FY1 on ward cover. You have just been bleeped about a 89-year-old with a background of metastatic prostate cancer. He is complaining of abdominal pain and the nurses would like you to administer some pain relief. They would also like you to prescribe some laxatives, as he has not opened his bowels for four days.

What are your differentials for this patient?

1. Related to metastatic prostate cancer:

   a. Hypercalcaemia (gives abdominal pain and constipation)
   b. Spinal metastases resulting in cord compression (urinary retention can cause pain)
   c. Urinary retention secondary to local prostate disease

2. Unrelated to metastatic prostate cancer:

   a. Surgical acute abdomen, i.e., bowel obstruction

How would you assess this patient?

I would follow the ALS approach and carry out a systematic primary survey using the A to E assessment.

A	If the patient is verbalising, I would assume that the airway is patent. I would like to put the patient on a 15L non-rebreathe mask.
B	I would like to check the sats and RR at this point. Consider an erect CXR is suspecting an acute abdomen.
C	Next, I would like to ensure the patient has good IV access and send blood for the following: FBC, UE, CRP, Clotting, Bone profile, Mg. I would like to obtain an ECG trace. I would like to ensure that a catheter is inserted for accurate urine output measurement.
D	I would like to assess the GCS, Pupils and perform a thorough neurological examination, focussing on the lower limbs to exclude cauda equina syndrome.

E	I would like to fully expose as appropriate and examine the following:
	• Abdomen: bladder distension? • PR exam: to assess anal tone and faecal loading

Which signs do you expect if the patient has cauda equina syndrome?

1. Neurolgical examination findings in lower limbs (usually lower motor neurone signs bilaterally):

Tone	Reduced
Power	Reduced
Reflexes	Reduced
Sensation	May be reduced if severe
Co-ordination	May be impaired due to weakness

2. Abdominal examination: distended bladder
3. PR exam: reduced/no peri-anal sensation and no anal tone

What is the definitive management of cauda equina syndrome?

To investigate, an urgent MRI whole spine is required to delineate the site of compression and potential cause.
  Management includes:

1. Urgent neurosurgical opinion to see if surgery is indicated.
2. Discussion with an oncologist, in this case, who will usually recommend either commencing the patient on dexamethasone or urgent radiotherapy.

Chapter 4   The Academic Interview

4.1 The Generic Approach to the Academic Interview

4.1.1 *Why is critical appraisal important?*

All AFP interviews will require critical appraisal skills to some degree, and this is a skill that is often tested in core and specialty training interviews. Depending on the AUoA, the critical appraisal station layout will vary very slightly, and it is important to check this information on the relevant websites. For London, you are usually provided with an abstract prior to your interview with 15 minutes of preparation time (and 15 minutes to prepare the clinical interview vignettes).

The figure below outlines the main steps involved in critical appraisal interview stations for the AFP.

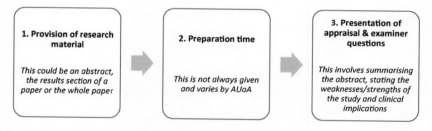

Key questions to be aware of when approaching any abstract/paper with example questions may include the following:

Critical Appraisal	What do you think of this paper/abstract?
	What are the strengths/weaknesses of this study?
	How could you improve the design of this study?
Statistical Definitions	Are the results significant?
	What is a p-value/confidence interval/statistical power?
Ethics	What are the ethical implications of this study?
Clinical Implications	How would you explain the result to patients?
	Should we change practice based on this research?

4.1.2 *How can I prepare for the academic interview?*

To prepare, you should practise appraising abstracts and answering mock examiner questions under timed conditions in small groups. To help with this, we have suggested a critical appraisal "checklist" in Section 4.3. Worked examples of appraised abstracts with questions are shown in Section 4.5. You should also refresh your knowledge about study design (Section 4.2), ethics (Section 4.4) and definitions of statistical terms (Section 4.6). Recommended reading and journals to source practice abstracts are listed in Section 4.7. Mock interviews are also included at the end of this book.

4.2 Types of Study Design and the Hierarchy of Evidence

The figure below outlines the hierarchy of evidence-based medicine. The strength of evidence increases as you move up the pyramid. It is important to be aware of this hierarchy and what each study design involves, including the main flaws. When approaching any paper/

abstract, it is important to be able to recognise which type of study design it follows in order to recognise the study's strengths/weaknesses.

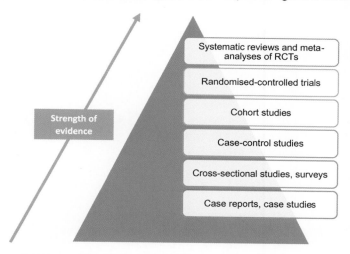

4.2.1 *Systematic reviews and meta-analyses*

A systematic review is a meticulous and protocol-driven literature review that integrates and critically analyses all published findings on a specific research question.

Meta-analysis is the statistical analysis of the results of several trials, which are combined in order to minimise bias, reach a more accurate "true" population effect, and increase the statistical power of the evidence. It is usually a part of systematic reviews. They may still be subject to publication bias because of differences between trials leading to some being excluded, and because of possible non-publication of trials with negative results.

You are less likely to encounter these types of studies at interviews, as they are often difficult to appraise. We would suggest not picking a systematic review for appraisal if you have the option of pre-preparing a paper.

4.2.2 *Randomised controlled trials, cohort and case-control studies*

Most interviews will provide you with either a randomised controlled trial (RCT), cohort study or a case-control study to analyse.

Randomised controlled trial	An experimental study where subjects are randomly allocated to either one of two arms of a study: Treatment A versus Treatment B or Treatment versus Placebo.

Pros	Cons
• Gold standard for studying treatment effects • Random allocation reduces selection bias and equally distributes confounding factors between treatment arms • Prospective: allows one to conclude causation between intervention and outcome • Reliably measures efficacy • Allows for meta-analyses	• Difficult • Time-consuming • Expensive • May be sponsored by pharmaceutical companies, introducing bias • May be prone to underpowering • Ethical problems in giving different treatments to the groups

Cohort study	An observational prospective study where groups are selected on the basis of their exposure to a particular agent (such as smoking tobacco). They are then followed over time to identify if they develop a particular outcome of interest (such as lung cancer). They can also be used to determine the prognosis of a disease (e.g., breast cancer is the exposure and death is the outcome).

Pros	Cons
• Can answer questions about aetiology and prognosis • Direct estimation of disease incidence rates • Can assess temporal relationships and causal links • Can assess multiple outcomes • Good for rare exposures • Can estimate risk ratios and odds ratios	• Can take a long time from exposure to measured outcomes • Cannot be used if diseases have long latency period • Expensive to set up and maintain • Bias is an issue if subjects drop out over time (often a large cohort is needed)

Case-control study

An observational retrospective study where patients can be divided into cases (people who have the disease in question) and controls (people without the disease). A relevant exposure is measured retrospectively and the frequency of exposure between the two groups is compared. This is quick, cheap and good for rare diseases, but is prone to recall bias.

Pros	Cons
• Good for studying rare diseases • Useful when there is a long latency period between a risk factor and outcome (as no waiting required) • Quick and cheap as few subjects required • Requires fewer patients	• Can be difficult to match to the control group • Rely on recall and records to identify risk factors (recall bias) • Temporal relationship difficult as subjects forget about sequence of events (symptom appearance) — relies on reverse causation

4.2.3 *Cross-sectional study*

This is where a representative sample population is recruited and then interviewed, examined or studied to gain answers to specific questions. Data is collected at a single time point but can refer retrospectively to health experiences in the past.

These are useful in estimating the prevalence of diseases and gaining an idea of the normal distribution for a population.

4.3 How to Critically Appraise an Abstract in 15 Minutes

We recommend that you develop a critical appraisal checklist, which you can apply to any abstract. Your checklist should include all the main components required to appraise a scientific article. If you practise using this checklist, you will become more confident and have a framework to fall back on during the stress of the interview.

We have provided an example of a 4-point checklist below. How you structure your appraisal is up to individual preference — you can adapt the checklist to suit yourself.

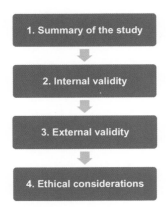

Note that the checklist is designed for randomised controlled trials, but can be adapted to cover other study designs. *Internal validity* refers to how trustworthy a study's findings are based on the methodology and how rigorously it is performed (i.e., to what extent does the study measure what it sets out to measure). *External validity* refers to generalisability (are the conditions and the population representative?) and applicability (cost effectiveness and benefit to care).

1. Summary of the Study	• State the design of the study.
	• Summarise using the PICO method:
	  — Population: sample size, patient group.
	  — Intervention.
	  — Control.
	  — Outcome(s): measured outcomes.
	• Brief summary of results.

2. Internal Validity	• State the **study design:**
	  — Mention its position on the hierarchy of evidence.
	  — Mention some pros and cons of using this design.
	• **Population:**
	  — Mention the recruitment method (check for selection bias).
	  — Mention sample size.
	    ▪ Comment that you would check a power calculation in the full text if relevant.
	  — Mention inclusion/exclusion criteria (check for selection bias).
	• **Intervention:**
	  — Examine if this is appropriate for the study question.
	  — If the study is a RCT, is blinding maintained (reduces observer bias)?
	• **Outcomes:**
	  — What are the endpoints used? Are they appropriate for the research question?
	    ▪ *Types of endpoints include primary, composite and surrogate.*
	  — Brief comment on statistics:
	    ▪ If the study is a RCT, was the data analysed per protocol or via the intention to treat the method (see glossary)?

	— Mention if the outcomes are designed *a priori*. 　▪ This means they were chosen before the study began, which prevents investigators selecting outcomes based on whether or not the result will be significant (known as "data dredging"); most studies with a trial registration number are designed *a priori*. — Comment on follow up time. • **Bias** (if not mentioned above): — Check for funding/conflict of interest declarations.
3. External Validity	External validity allows you to answer the question: "Will this study change clinical practice?" Broadly speaking, you will need to discuss the study's generalisability and applicability: • **Generalisability:** 　○ Where was the study conducted (ranging from single centre to global)? 　○ Is the patient population representative? • **Applicability:** 　○ Are the study resources available in most settings? 　○ Cost effectiveness and benefit to care (number needed to treat for the study intervention). Ultimately, you should say: "I would read the full paper and seek further evidence, ideally in the form of a systematic review +/– meta-analysis."
4. Ethical Considerations	You should include a brief comment on ethical issues raised by the study (see Section 4.4).

4.4 Research Ethics

In your answer, think about the following with respect to medical ethics:

- Type of study:
  - For example, is it ethical to randomise people to a treatment that could be less effective than the study intervention?
- Population:
  - Are they able to give informed consent?
- Outcomes:
  - For example, use of interim analyses to halt trials if interventions are already shown to be significantly harmful/beneficial.
- Investigators/authors:
  - Are they biased in any way, e.g., from funding?
- Generalisability:
  - If approved, would the study intervention be available for everyone?

Key terms to be aware of:

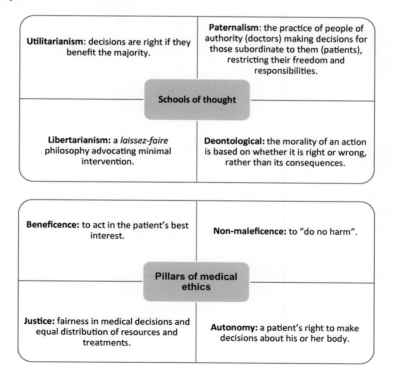

4.5 Examples of Critically Appraising the Most Commonly Encountered Studies

In this section, we provide worked examples for the following commonly encountered abstracts in the critical appraisal station:

- Medical randomised-controlled trial
- Surgical randomised-controlled trial
- Cohort study
- Case-control study

Abstract 1: Medical Randomised-Controlled Trial[1]

BACKGROUND

Point-of-care testing of C-reactive protein (CRP) may be a way to reduce unnecessary use of antibiotics without harming patients who have acute exacerbations of chronic obstructive pulmonary disease (COPD).

METHODS

We performed a multi-centre, open-label, randomised, controlled trial involving patients with a diagnosis of COPD in their primary care clinical record, who consulted a clinician at 1 of the 86 general medical practices in England and Wales for an acute exacerbation of COPD. The patients were assigned to receive usual care guided by CRP point-of-care testing (CRP-guided group) or usual care alone (usual-care group). The primary outcomes were: (1) patient-reported use of antibiotics for acute exacerbations of COPD within four weeks after randomisation (to show superiority) and (2) COPD-related health status at two weeks after randomisation, as measured by the Clinical COPD Questionnaire, a 10-item scale with scores ranging from 0 (very good COPD health status) to 6 (extremely poor COPD health status) to show non-inferiority.

RESULTS

A total of 653 patients underwent randomisation. Fewer patients in the CRP-guided group reported antibiotic use than in the usual-care group (57.0% versus 77.4%; adjusted odds ratio, 0.31; 95% confidence interval [CI], 0.20 to 0.47). The adjusted mean difference in the total

Abstract 1: (*Continued*)

score on the Clinical COPD Questionnaire at two weeks was −0.19 points (two-sided 90% CI, −0.33 to −0.05) in favor of the CRP-guided group. The antibiotic prescribing decisions made by clinicians at the initial consultation were ascertained for all but one patient — prescriptions issued over the first four weeks of follow-up accounted for 96.9% of the patients. A lower percentage of patients in the CRP-guided group than in the usual-care group received an antibiotic prescription at the initial consultation (47.7% versus 69.7%, for a difference of 22.0 percentage points; adjusted odds ratio, 0.31; 95% CI, 0.21 to 0.45) and during the first 4 weeks of follow-ups (59.1% versus 79.7%, for a difference of 20.6 percentage points; adjusted odds ratio, 0.30; 95% CI, 0.20 to 0.46). Two patients in the usual-care group died within four weeks after randomisation from causes considered by the investigators to be unrelated to trial participation.

CONCLUSIONS

CRP-guided prescribing of antibiotics for exacerbations of COPD in primary care clinics resulted in a lower percentage of patients who reported antibiotic use and who received antibiotic prescriptions from clinicians, with no evidence of harm. (Funded by the National Institute for Health Research Health Technology Assessment Program; PACE Current Controlled Trials number, ISRCTN24346473.)

Abstract 1: Critical Appraisal

1. Summary of the Study	• **Design:** This is a multi-centre, open label, randomised controlled trial. • **Population:** 653 patients with a diagnosis of COPD in their primary care record who consulted a GP in England and Wales for an acute exacerbation of COPD. • **Intervention:** use of CRP point-of-care testing • **Control:** usual care • **Outcome(s):** patient-reported use of antibiotics within four weeks post randomisation;

	COPD-related health status within two weeks post randomisation. • **Summary of findings:** CRP-guided prescribing of antibiotics for exacerbations of COPD in primary care resulted in less antibiotic use and no evidence of harm.
2. Internal Validity	**Study design:** • This is a multi-centre, open label, randomised controlled trial, which is high on the hierarchy of evidence and reduces selection bias; it is open label, however, it would be very difficult to ethically "blind" this intervention. **Population:** • Recruitment (GP visit): this excludes more severe cases in hospital. • Large sample (n = 653): it would be important to check the power calculation in the full text. • Inclusion/exclusion criteria: limited information on this; not all COPD exacerbations are infective. **Intervention:** • It would be important to find out *how* exactly CRP testing was used to guide treatment. • The intervention was not blinded — this would be very difficult.
	Outcomes: • The outcomes were likely designed *a priori*, suggested by the clinical trials registry number, which reduces "data dredging". • Patient-reported use of antibiotics is an outcome prone to recall bias. • COPD-related health status at two weeks is a good holistic/safety outcome.

	• The follow-up time is relatively short (2–4 weeks) for a chronic condition with (often) recurrent exacerbations.
	Statistics:
	• Unclear if the results were analysed using an intention to treat or per protocol approach (the full text should be checked for this).
	• The attrition rate was low, which reduces exclusion bias.
3. External Validity	• The study was multi-centre but limited to England and Wales.
	• No data was presented on cost-effectiveness.
	• Point-of-care CRP tests are not routine/available in all GP practices or hospitals.
	⇒ This study is important because COPD exacerbations are common and do not always need to be treated with antibiotics. Moreover, antibiotic use incurs cost, potential for side effects and contributes to resistance.
	⇒ I would like to read the full paper and ideally offer a systematic review ± meta-analysis on this topic.
4. Ethics	• This study raises ethical issues related to the principles of beneficence/non-maleficence. Patients in the intervention arm who were not given antibiotics may have received them in the control arm (this could have caused harm because point-of-care CRP testing was not validated when the study began).

Example Questions	
1. What are the strengths and weaknesses of this study design?	Refer to the pros and cons of randomised controlled trials.

Example Questions	
2. Define 95% confidence intervals	The range in which the population value will lie 95% of the time. For significance, if the result is an absolute difference, the confidence interval cannot cross 0. If the result is a ratio, the confidence interval cannot cross 1.
3. Are the results statistically significant? Why?	For ratios (risk ratio, odds ratio), the result is significant if the confidence interval does not cross 1. For absolute values (e.g., scores on a questionnaire), the result is significant if the confidence interval does not cross 0.
4. Should point-of-care CRP tests be used routinely?	This is a personal judgment call, and if you substantiate your answer you will not be criticised. It is a good idea to mention that you would ideally like to review further studies and stronger evidence on this topic in the form of a systematic review ± meta-analysis (if available).
5. How would you explain the study result to patients?	In GP practices, a point-of-care test that measures a marker of infection/inflammation can be used to help doctors decide who can safely avoid antibiotic treatment for exacerbations of their COPD.

Abstract 2: Surgical Randomised-controlled Trial[2]

BACKGROUND

The timing and indications for surgical intervention in asymptomatic patients with severe aortic stenosis remain controversial.

METHODS

In a multi-centre trial, we randomly assigned 145 asymptomatic patients with very severe aortic stenosis (defined as an aortic-valve area of ≤ 0.75 cm^2 with either an aortic jet velocity of ≥ 4.5 m per second or

Abstract 2: (*Continued*)

a mean transaortic gradient of ≥50 mm Hg) to early surgery or conservative care, according to the recommendations of current guidelines. The primary endpoint was a composite of death during or within 30 days after surgery (often called operative mortality) or death from cardiovascular causes during the entire follow-up period. The major secondary endpoint was death from any cause during a follow-up.

RESULTS

In the early surgery group, 69 of 73 patients (95%) underwent surgery within 2 months after randomisation, and there was no operative mortality. In an intention-to-treat analysis, a primary endpoint event occurred in 1 patient in the early surgery group (1%) and in 11 of the 72 patients in the conservative care group (15%) (hazard ratio, 0.09; 95% confidence interval [CI], 0.01 to 0.67; $P = 0.003$). Death from any cause occurred in 5 patients in the early surgery group (7%) and 15 patients in the conservative care group (21%) (hazard ratio, 0.33; 95% CI, 0.12 to 0.90). In the conservative care group, the cumulative incidence of sudden death was 4% at four years and 14% at eight years.

CONCLUSIONS

Among asymptomatic patients with very severe aortic stenosis, the incidence of the composite of operative mortality or death from cardiovascular causes during the follow-up period was significantly lower among those who underwent early aortic-valve replacement surgery than among those who received conservative care. (Funded by the Korean Institute of Medicine; RECOVERY ClinicalTrials.gov number, NCT01161732.)

Abstract 2: Critical Appraisal

1. Summary of the Study	• **Design:** This is a multi-centre randomised controlled trial. • **Population:** 145 asymptomatic patients with very severe aortic stenosis.

	• **Intervention:** Early aortic valve replacement surgery. • **Control:** Conservative management. • **Outcome(s):** The primary outcome was a composite of death during or within 30 days of surgery or death from cardiovascular causes during the entire follow-up period; the secondary outcome was death from any cause during a follow-up. • **Summary of findings:** In patients with asymptomatic but very severe aortic stenosis, early surgical intervention is associated with lower mortality than conservative management.
2. Internal Validity	**Study design:** • This is a multi-centre randomised controlled trial, which is high on the hierarchy of evidence and reduces selection bias. **Population:** • Moderately sized sample (n = 145); it would be important to check the power calculation in the full text. • Inclusion/exclusion criteria: the definition of severe aortic stenosis is clearly defined, which allows for reproducibility. It would be important to check how the authors defined "asymptomatic" — was this patient reported or were criteria formed? Given that aortic stenosis occurs in older patients, it would be important to check the baseline demographics of both groups for comorbidities, which could affect the results. **Intervention:** • The intervention was early aortic valve replacement; this is an invasive surgery that might not be appropriate for less surgically fit patients, therefore potentially introducing selection bias.

Outcomes:

- The primary outcome was a composite of operative mortality (within 30 days after surgery) and cardiovascular death during the follow-up period (eight years). Composite outcomes have increased statistical efficiency (i.e., require fewer endpoints to reach statistical significance) but are more difficult to interpret. The follow-up period is, however, sufficiently long to determine the long-term effects of surgery and outcomes of conservative management.
- The outcomes were likely determined *a priori* (clinical trials number included in the abstract), which has the advantage of reducing data dredging.
- Outcomes such as "death from cardiovascular causes" or "death during follow-up" are prone to confounding, particularly in a population with severe aortic stenosis. Patients are likely to be older and may have multiple (potentially cardiac) comorbidities.
- Additionally, no patient-reported or functional outcomes are described in the abstract; it would be important to check the full-text for any patient-reported symptomatic improvements post-surgery.

Statistics:

- An intention-to-treat analysis was used, which means that all subjects randomised to the treatment arms were included in the final analyses with the advantage of mirroring "real life" practice.
- It would be important to find out why 5% of patients allocated to early surgery did not undergo surgery within two months of randomisation, and also to read the full descriptions of the primary and secondary endpoints that occurred.

3. External Validity	• The study was multi-centre, which increases its generalisability. • The study reporting would benefit from a cost effectiveness analysis or number needed to treat calculation with respect to early surgery preventing deaths. ⇒ This study is important because aortic stenosis is a common, potentially fatal condition, and there is clinical equipoise regarding the benefits of early surgery in asymptomatic patients. However, the study abstract does not discuss all the important factors to consider in management decisions, including surgical fitness and patient choice. One way in which this research could be practice-changing is if the results are discussed with patients to help them make informed management decisions. Ideally, I would like to read the full paper and perform a systematic review ± meta-analysis on this topic.
4. Ethics	• Ethical issues to consider in this abstract include: ⇒ Beneficence/non-maleficence: patients randomised to the control arm had a higher mortality rate; this harm could have been minimised with an interval safety analysis. On the contrary, from a utilitarian perspective, it could be argued that the study is ethically justified because the findings will go on to benefit many more future patients by confirming that early surgery has a survival benefit. ⇒ Autonomy: in randomised controlled trials, patients have no choice as to which treatment arm they are allocated. However, they can drop out if they wish.

⇒ Justice: it would be important to consider if the study intervention (early aortic valve surgery) is available for eligible patients in all settings, including those where healthcare is rationed (e.g., the NHS).

	Example Questions
1. What is a composite outcome? What are the advantages and disadvantages of composite outcomes?	Composite outcomes have multiple combined endpoints. They are often used in randomised controlled trials because they are more efficient, i.e., fewer endpoints are required for statistical significance. The main disadvantage of composite outcomes is that they are difficult to interpret (i.e., you cannot tell which of the composites is driving the overall result). Another disadvantage is that it is often difficult for researchers to decide which outcomes should be included in the composite outcome.
2. Explain what an intention-to-treat analysis is and the advantages of this method. What is an alternative to an intention-to-treat analysis?	An intention-to-treat analysis means that all subjects randomised are included in the analyses as members of the groups they were initially allocated to, regardless of whether they completed the study. This means that people who drop out due to, for example, side effects or inefficacy, are still included and therefore the results mirror "real life" practice. In a per protocol analysis, only data from those subjects who complied with the trial protocol through to completion are considered in the analysis. This has the advantages of showing the "true" treatment effect when the intervention is administered as per the

Example Questions	
	protocol but does not account for patients who drop out because they fail to improve or have intolerable side effects. Per protocol analyses are therefore prone to exclusion bias.
	Both types of analysis can be useful and appropriate depending on the research question. In general, intention-to-treat analyses are preferable in clinical studies because the findings are more realistic.
3. Define "hazard ratio"	The hazard ratio can be defined as the hazard rate of the experimental arm divided by the control arm, where the hazard rate is the probability of an endpoint occurring in a set time interval, divided by the duration of that time interval.
4. Define "p-value"	The probability of getting the observed results by chance. When p is less than the alpha level (often set at 0.05), the results are statistically significant.

Abstract 3: Cohort Study[3]

BACKGROUND

Chemotherapy for metastatic lung or colorectal cancer can prolong life by weeks or months and may provide palliation, but it is not curative.

METHODS

We studied 1,193 patients participating in the Cancer Care Outcomes Research and Surveillance (CanCORS) study (a national, prospective, observational cohort study). These participants were still alive four months after diagnosis and received chemotherapy for their metastatic (stage IV) lung or colorectal cancer. We sought to characterise the prevalence of the expectation that chemotherapy might be curative and to identify the clinical, sociodemographic, and health-system factors associated with this expectation. Data was obtained from a patient survey by professional interviewers in addition to a comprehensive review of medical records.

Abstract 3: (*Continued*)

RESULTS

Overall, 69% of patients with lung cancer and 81% of those with colorectal cancer did not understand that chemotherapy was not at all likely to cure their cancer. In multi-variable logistic regression, the risk of reporting inaccurate beliefs about chemotherapy was higher among patients with colorectal cancer, as compared to those with lung cancer (odds ratio, 1.75; 95% confidence interval [CI], 1.29 to 2.37); among non-white and Hispanic patients, as compared with non-Hispanic white patients (odds ratio for Hispanic patients, 2.82; 95% CI, 1.51 to 5.27; odds ratio for black patients, 2.93; 95% CI, 1.80 to 4.78); and among patients who rated their communication with their physician very favourably, as compared with less favourably (odds ratio for highest third vs. lowest third, 1.90; 95% CI, 1.33 to 2.72). The educational level, functional status, and the patient's role in decision-making were not associated with such inaccurate beliefs about chemotherapy.

CONCLUSIONS

Many patients receiving chemotherapy for incurable cancers may not understand that chemotherapy is unlikely to be curative, which could compromise their ability to make informed treatment decisions that are consonant with their preferences. Physicians may be able to improve patients' understanding, but this may come at the cost of patients' satisfaction with them. (Funded by the National Cancer Institute and others.)

Abstract 3: Critical Appraisal

1. Summary of the Study	• **Design:** This was an observational study looking at characterising the prevalence of the expectation that chemotherapy might be curative, and to identify the clinical, sociodemographic and health-system factors associated with this expectation. • **Population:** 1,193 patients participating in CanCORS and receiving chemotherapy for metastatic stage 4 lung or colorectal cancer.

	Summary of findings: • The study found that many patients receiving chemotherapy for incurable cancers may not realise that the chemotherapy is unlikely to be curative, particularly in patients with colorectal cancer, who are non-white and Hispanic, and who rate communication with their doctor highly.
2. Internal Validity	**Study design:** • This was an observational study, which is the most appropriate for observing trends and collecting epidemiological data. **Population:** • Recruitment: the recruited patients were already participating in a study, so they were more likely to look after their health, see the benefit of research, and educate themselves about treatment (membership bias). However, the study was national and prospective, with a wide catchment, which reduces selection bias compared to other forms of sampling. • Sample size: large (>1,000 patients); it would be important to check the full text to see if the study was adequately powered. • Inclusion criteria: included patients were alive four months after diagnosis and receiving chemotherapy for lung/colorectal cancer; this out-selects people with faster growing tumours who may have a better idea of their palliative status (Neyman/ survival bias). **Intervention:** • Some factors to consider regarding the patient survey administered by professional interviewers:

- Was the survey validated?
- Did it use language that patients could understand?
- Was the survey piloted?
- Who recorded the answers of the survey? If done by doctors, this could have resulted in bias results in favour of the expected outcome.
- Patients may not recall accurately information given to them by doctors (recall bias).

- Regarding the review of medical records, it is possible that some data was missing.

Outcomes:

- It is not entirely clear how/if certain terms were explained to patients, for example "not at all likely to cure cancer"; an alternative would be to ask patients how long they thought chemotherapy would be able to prolong their lives.
- It is unclear from the abstract which aspects of communications with doctors were rated.
- It would be important to know how educational status stratified and if a validated measure of functional status was used.

Statistics:

- Multi-variate logistic regression was used; this has the advantage of adjusting for confounders.

3. External Validity	- National study - Unclear what patient demographics were and if this is applicable to patients of all cancer aetiologies.

4. Ethics	• Ethical issues to consider in this abstract include:
	⇒ Autonomy versus Paternalism: important to provide all the information to allow for informed decision-making but this may risk physician-patient rapport.

Example Questions	
1. What are the strengths and weaknesses of this study design?	State pros and cons of cohort studies, as per Section 4.2
2. Define "odds ratio".	Ratio of the odds of the outcome occurring in the experimental group vs. control group.
3. Define "bias". What types of bias could apply to this study?	Bias relates to any factor, which impacts the study result in a non-random way, such that the result is not a true result. Types of bias which could affect this study: • Membership bias: the included patients are already participating in a study so might be more likely to look after their health, see the benefit of research, and educate themselves about treatment; • Neyman/survival bias and selection bias: included patients had to be alive four months after diagnosis and receiving chemotherapy; this out-selects people with faster growing tumours who may have a more realistic idea of their palliative status; • Recall bias: affects any study in which questionnaires are used to elicit information.

Abstract 4: Case-control Study[4]

BACKGROUND

Dupuytren's disease is a complex condition, with both genetic and environmental factors contributing to its aetiology. We aimed to quantify the extent to which genetic factors predispose to the disease, through the calculation of the sibling recurrence risk (ls), and to calculate the proportion of heritability accounted for by the currently known genetic loci.

METHODS

From 174 siblings of patients with surgically confirmed disease, 100 were randomly selected. Controls were recruited from patients attending an ophthalmology outpatient clinic for eye conditions unrelated to diabetes.

RESULTS

There were no statistically significant differences in baseline characteristics between the case and control groups. In siblings, 47% had Dupuytren's disease, compared with 10% of the controls, giving a sibling recurrence risk (ls) of 4.5. The currently known loci that are predisposed to Dupuytren's disease account for 12.1% of the total heritability of the disease.

CONCLUSION

Dupuytren's disease was significantly more common in siblings than in controls. These results accurately quantify the magnitude of the genetic predisposition to Dupuytren's disease.

Abstract 4: Critical Appraisal

1. Summary of the Study	• **Design:** This is a case-control study. • **Population (cases):** 100 siblings of the surgically confirmed disease. • **Control:** 124 patients attending an ophthalmology outpatient clinic. • **Outcome:** Sibling recurrence risk; proportion of total heritability from the currently known loci. • **Summary of findings:** Dupuytren's disease is significantly more common in siblings (by about 4.5 times).

2. Internal Validity	**Study design:**
	• This study was a case-control design, which is appropriate for answering this research question.
	• The advantages of this research study design are that it is quicker, cheaper, requires fewer patients and does not require a latency period to determine a link between risk factors and outcomes (as cohort studies do). However, it can be difficult to match cases and controls well.
	Population:
	• Index patients had previous surgery, and therefore the investigators may have recruited siblings from a skewed sample with a more severe disease.
	• Controls were recruited from ophthalmology outpatient clinics for non-diabetic eye conditions, which is a positive because there are no currently known shared genetic or environmental risk factors for Dupuytren's and non-diabetic eye disease.
	• The full text would need to be scrutinised to ensure that adequate demographic information was collected for the purposes of matching, i.e., age, gender, ethnicity, diabetes, alcohol intake (confounders), past surgery (marker of disease severity).
	Outcomes:
	• The outcomes are focused and appropriate for the study question. Additional secondary outcomes to check for in the full text include the risk of Dupuytren's disease based on sex, age and past history of surgery.

3. External Validity	• The prevalence of Dupuytren's disease differs geographically; it would be important to know where the research participants were recruited. ⇒ Dupuytren's disease is a complex condition with genetic and environmental influences. Its pathophysiology is largely unknown, so it is important to quantify the extent to which genetics contributes. More knowledge about genetic architecture could lead to rational designs of new therapies.

Example Questions	
1. What are the strengths and weaknesses of this study design?	State the pros and cons of case-control studies, Section 4.2.
2. Define "confounder" and list some confounding factors that would need to be controlled in this study.	A confounder has a triangular relationship between the exposure and outcome but is not on the causal pathway. It might make it appear as if there is a direct relationship between the exposure and outcome (positive confounder) or mask an association that would have been present (negative confounder). Possible confounders in this study include age, ethnicity, comorbidities (diabetes mellitus, alcohol intake), past surgery, previous family history, drug history, etc.

4.6 Critical Appraisal Glossary[5,6]

Term	Definition
Statistical Terms	
Evidence-based medicine	The conscientious, explicit and judicious use of current best evidence in making decisions about the care of individual patients.
Confidence interval	The range in which the population value will lie 95% of the time. If the result is an absolute difference: CI cannot cross 0. If the result is RR or OR: CI cannot cross 1.
Number needed to treat	The number of subjects who must be treated with the intervention, compared to the control, for one additional subject to experience the beneficial outcome (1/ARR), where ARR = absolute risk reduction.
Hazard rate	The probability of an endpoint in a time interval divided by the duration of the time interval.
Hazard ratio	The hazard rate of the experimental arm divided by the control arm.
Confounder	A confounder has a triangular relationship between the exposure and outcome but is not on the causal pathway. It makes it appear as if there is a direct relationship between the exposure and outcome (positive confounder) or might mask an association that would have been present (negative confounder).
Per protocol analysis	Only data from those subjects who complied with trial protocol through to completion are considered in the analysis. • Advantages: shows the true treatment effect, shows how things are when processes are completed.

Term	Definition
	Statistical Terms
	• Disadvantages: patients not accounted for may have failed to improve, or had intolerable side effects and dropped out (exclusion bias).

Intention to treat analysis	All subjects randomised are included in the analyses as members of the groups they were allocated, regardless of whether they completed the study.
	
	 • Advantages: mirrors real life practice.
	 • Methods for dealing with missing data:
	  ○ Worst-case scenario.
	  ○ Hot deck imputation: fill in missing values from similar subjects with complete records.
	  ○ Last observation carried forward.

Absolute risk (%)	Incidence rate of the outcome = outcome in either control or experimental arm/total number of participants in arm.
Absolute risk reduction (%)	Risk in controls — risk in experimental group.
Relative risk	Experimental event rate (EER) or risk/control event rate (CER) or risk • =1: no difference • >1: increased risk • <1: decreased risk
Relative risk reduction	Reduction in risk in control group vs. experimental group/risk in control group • = CER-EER/CER

Term	Definition
Statistical Terms	
Odds ratio	Ratio of the odds of outcome occurring in experimental group vs. control group • Used in cross-sectional and case-control studies. • **NB:** Log odds ratio is not significant if CI crosses 0, not 1.
Null hypothesis	The assumption that any difference between experimental groups is due to chance.
P-value	The probability of getting the observed results by chance. When p is greater than the alpha level, the results are statistically significant.
Type 1 error	False positive, wrongful rejection of null hypothesis = alpha. Due to bias, confounding, data dredging.
Type 2 error	False negative, wrongful acceptance of null hypothesis = beta = 1–alpha. Due to the sample size being too small or measurement variance being too large.
Power	The probability that a type 2 error will not be made in the study, i.e., the study's ability to detect the smallest possible difference between the groups that is considered clinically worthwhile. 0.8 is adequate (80% chance of finding significant difference, if a difference exists).

Study Phases	
Phase I Clinical trial	These are "first in human" studies usually conducted on a small number of healthy volunteers to determine the tolerability and safety of a new drug, as well as its pharmacokinetics and pharmacodynamics.

Study Phases	
Phase II Clinical trial	These are "dose-finding" trials usually on patients — a lower number than Phase III but larger than Phase I — assessing optimal dosing (giving different doses and following up to determine the efficacy and tolerability/toxicity) and efficacy (biological effect of the drug).
Phase III Clinical trial	These trials assess the effectiveness of a new drug/intervention, as compared to the gold standard therapy (whilst always ensuring its safety), to inform the value of the new intervention in clinical practice. They are usually multi-centre randomised control trials on large numbers of patients.
Post-marketing surveillance (Phase IV)	Monitors safety of the drug after it is being marketed (pharmacovigilance), to detect any rare or long-term adverse events or side effects that were not detected during the previous trials.

Study Design	
Randomisation	The process of assigning trial subjects to treatment or control groups using an element of chance, so that each participant has an equal chance of being allocated to either group. This is to reduce allocation bias and balance known and unknown possible confounding factors, such that any difference between the two groups is purely by chance.
Stratified randomisation	Prevents imbalance between treatment groups for known factors that influence prognosis or treatment responsiveness. As a result, stratification may prevent type I error and improve power for small trials (<400 patients), but only when the stratification factors have a large effect on the prognosis.

Study Design	
Allocation concealment	Refers to masking the randomisation code or sequence before patients are recruited, so that investigators don't know what group the next patient will be randomised to, thus avoiding selection bias.
Blinding	Involves masking the allocation of the treatment group after randomisation, so one or more parties involved in the trial are not aware whether the participants are in the intervention or the control group. This aims to remove bias, including performance and observer bias.
Efficacy	The capacity for the therapeutic effect of a given intervention, e.g., whether a drug demonstrates a health benefit over a placebo or other intervention when tested in an ideal situation. These are called explanatory trials.
Effectiveness	How well an intervention works in practice, i.e., in the real world outside a clinical trial. This tends to be lower than the efficacy. These are called pragmatic trials.
Placebo	Traditionally refers to a substance or treatment with no active therapeutic effect. In medical research, it is unethical to give a substance without therapeutic effect when one is available. Hence, a placebo refers to the control used, for example, the gold-standard intervention in which the intervention of interest is being measured against.
Surrogate endpoint	A variable that is relatively easily measured and which predicts a rare or distant outcome of the intervention tested. It is not a direct measure of either harm or clinical benefit.

Bias	
Selection bias	There is a problem with the way the subjects are recruited and allocated to groups. The sample population is unrepresentative of the target population.
Diagnostic purity bias	Comorbidity is excluded in the sample population, such that it does not reflect the true complexity of cases in the population.
Neyman bias (survival bias)	There is a time gap between the onset of a condition and the selection of the study population, such that some individuals with the condition are not available for selection.
Response bias	Individuals volunteer for studies but they differ some way from the target population, e.g., they are more motivated to improve health.
Lead-time bias	Screening/testing increases the perceived survival time without affecting the course of the disease.
Publication bias	A study that shows a significant difference between two interventions is more likely to be published than a negative study.
Observation bias	There is a problem with the way data is collected in the study, such that the data has been unduly influenced by the expectations of the researchers and subjects.
Response bias	The subject answers questions in the way in which they think the researcher wants them to answer, e.g., subjects in the experimental arm are more likely to give favourable responses.
Recall bias	Subjects selectively remember details from the past.

Bias	
Exclusion bias	Results from differences in dropout rates between groups.
Hawthorne effect	Subjects alter their behaviour because they are aware they are being observed in a study.
Performance bias	Differences in care provided aside from intervention.
Detection bias	Differences in how outcomes are assessed between groups.

Ethics	
Declaration of Helsinki	New treatments should be tested against the current best treatment, except when no proven treatment exists, or for compelling/scientifically sound reasons, the use of a placebo is necessary, and patients will not be at risk of serious/irreversible harm.

4.7 Useful Resources

Books
- *How to Read a Paper* — Trisha Greenhalgh
- *The Doctor's Guide to Critical Appraisal* — Narinder Gosall and Gurpal Gosall

Journals
- *New England Journal of Medicine*
- *The Lancet*
- *The BMJ*

4.8 References

1. Butler CC, Gillespie D, White P, *et al.* (2019) C-reactive protein testing to guide antibiotic prescribing for COPD exacerbations. *N Eng J Med* **381**(2): 111–20.

2. Kang D-H, Park S-J, Lee S-A, *et al.* (2019) Early surgery or conservative care for asymptomatic aortic stenosis. *N Eng J Med* **382**(2): 111–9.
3. Weeks JC, Catalano PJ, Cronin A, *et al.* (2012) Patients' expectations about effects of chemotherapy for advanced cancer, *N Engl J Med* **367**(17): 1616–25.
4. Capstick R, Bragg T, Giele H, Furniss D. (2012) Sibling recurrence risk in Dupuytren's disease, *J Hand Surg* **38**(4): 424–9.
5. Gosall N, Gosall G. (2015) *The Doctor's Guide to Critical Appraisal*, 4th ed. PasTest.
6. Greenhalgh T. (2010) *How to Read a Paper: The Basics of Evidence-Based Medicine*, 4th ed. Wiley-Blackwell.

Chapter
5
Mock Interview Stations

In the following section, we will provide four mock clinical stations and four mock academic interview stations. We suggest that you combine a clinical interview example with an academic one and practice these under timed conditions.

These mock stations are by no means a complete representation of all the scenarios that may arise; you may find it beneficial to write some vignettes of your own, once you become familiar with the pattern and style of questions commonly used.

Finally, always consult the latest guidelines alongside local guidelines for each of the following clinical scenarios; the mock answers and explanations provided here are for guidance only. Ensure you follow the full recommendations outlined in Chapters 3 and 4.

5.1 Exemplar Mark Schemes

We have created the following marking schemes for each of the interview stations, which you can use as a reference. Please also note that the marking scheme used in this section was written by the authors and is intended to cover the key components assessed in most interviews. It does not necessarily reflect the marking scheme used in any particular deanery.

Academic Interview Mark Scheme

Domain	5 – Outstanding 4 – Excellent 3 – Good 2 – Adequate 1 – Unsatisfactory 0 – Unanswered
1. Evidence of interest in Academic Medicine *The candidate should be able to give reasons for choosing to pursue academic medicine and demonstrate an awareness of the academic field (e.g., the ACF, PhDs, etc.).*	
2. Ability to provide a holistic understanding of the abstract *The candidate should be able to understand why the study was done, what its key findings were, and be able to place the research in its context.*	
3. Ability to interpret the results of the abstract *The candidate should be able to interpret the statistics and results of the study and summarise these in a way that could be understood by patients.*	
4. Ability to identify weaknesses in the study *This includes the ability of the candidate to identify sources of bias, confounding, and other flaws in the methodology.*	
5. Understanding of research ethics *The candidate should be aware of the process of obtaining ethical approval and be able to identify potential ethical issues that may have arisen during the designing of this study.*	

6. Ability to suggest further research avenues based on the findings of this study	
7. Ability to communicate effectively with the examiner *The candidate should be able to succinctly and effectively summarise their findings. They should be able to establish rapport with the interviewers, and answer questions directly and appropriately.*	
Total:	

Clinical Interview Mark Scheme

Domain	5 – Outstanding 4 – Excellent 3 – Good 2 – Adequate 1 – Unsatisfactory 0 – Unanswered
1. Ability to interpret and prioritise the clinical scenarios *The candidate should be able to prioritise the sickest patients and be able to justify which patient they will attend to first.*	
2. Ability to conduct a thorough and safe A to E assessment *The candidate should offer to take a brief, focused history, before demonstrating a systematic understanding of the A to E approach and be able to apply this to the patient. They are aware of when to progress through each stage of the assessment.*	

3. Ability to request and interpret clinical results *The candidate should be able to suggest relevant tests and interpret results from basic investigations such as ABGs and blood tests.*	
4. Ability to work within the limits of their confidence *The candidate is aware of when they should ask for other help, including the assistance of seniors. The candidate demonstrates safe practice at all times.*	
5. Clinical knowledge and management of emergency scenarios *The candidate should demonstrate sound clinical knowledge, in keeping with that of an FY1 doctor. They should be able to confidently suggest initial management of patients and be aware of appropriate escalation measures.*	
6. Ability to communicate effectively with the examiner *The candidate should be able to succinctly and effectively summarise their findings. They should also be able to establish rapport with the interviewers, and answer questions directly and appropriately.*	
Total:	

5.2 Clinical Interview Stations

Mock Clinical Station 1

You are an FY1 in respiratory medicine, working at a busy District General Hospital. You have just stopped at Costa to buy your favourite Christmas-themed drink when the following occurs:

1. You receive a bleep from a nurse in Ward A asking you to see James, a 23-year-old man who is becoming increasingly breathless. He was admitted yesterday morning following an asthma attack, and the nurse is concerned because his breathing is deteriorating despite having received two puffs of salbutamol. She says that he cannot complete sentences when they were having a conversation about Coronavirus and its economic implications.

2. You receive a bleep from a nurse in Ward B who would like you to review a 51-year-old patient with known alcoholic hepatitis and no other previous medical history. This patient is sweating and appears slightly agitated. The nurses state he is more tremulous than usual. His RR is 20, sats 99% on room air, BP is 128/80, and HR is 88.

3. You receive a WhatsApp message from your registrar, who says that there is a lumbar puncture that is going to be performed, and they want to observe you performing it so that you can develop your skills. The procedure will be performed in 5 minutes.

4. You walk past the reception desk of Ward C, where your cousins are waiting to receive an update about your great aunt's health. She is a patient of Ward C. They are becoming increasingly distressed since they are not updated, especially since you are a part of the family.

How will you proceed?

Suggested questions:

- Which patient would you attend to first and why?
- Outline your approach to these scenarios.
- What are the most likely differentials for each of these patients?
- What are you most concerned about in each of the vignettes?

1. Emphasise that safety of patients is a priority	Safety of patients is the main priority. Therefore, I would prioritise patients who are most unwell. In this case the main issues are: 1. Breathing problem in patient 1 2. D problem (delirium tremens) in patient 2

	3. Distressed relatives in scenario 4 4. Developing clinical skills in scenario 3 Based on this, I believe patient 1 is the most unwell, followed by patient 2. I would then address the relatives of patient 4.
2. Make seniors aware if there are more than 1 unwell patient	I would text my registrar back to let him know that I have 2 unwell patients and will not be able to make it in time to perform the lumbar puncture.
3. Get the nurses to carry out investigations on the other patients in the meantime, if necessary	Whilst I go to assess patient 1, I would like to advise the nurses to do the following for patient 2: • Take blood: FBC, UE, CRP, Clotting, Crossmatch • Site a cannula • ECG trace • Monitor urine output • Regular observations and escalate if further deterioration. • **CIWA** score him (important for tailoring treatment of alcohol withdrawal).

4. State the most worrying concerns for each of the patients with a brief list of differentials	• **Patient 1:** most likely has an exacerbation of Asthma.
	  ○ Other differentials: Pneumonia, Pneumothorax.
	• **Patient 2:** most likely has EtOH withdrawal, I would be most worried about risk of seizures secondary to this.
	  ○ Other differentials: hepatic encephalopathy, infection (meningitis/encephalitis), electrolyte disturbances, or substance misuse.

5. Carry out the A to E assessment for the first patient	I would like to assess **patient 1** first. I would follow the ALS approach and carry out a systematic primary survey using the A to E assessment.

Go through the A to E assessment as outlined in Chapter 3 but remember to tailor it to this case specifically. You can do this by outlining the features of severe and life-threatening asthma.

Moderate	Severe	Life-threatening
Peak flow >50–75% predicted	Peak flow 33–50% best	Peak flow <33%
	RR >25%	SpO$_2$ <92%
	HR >110	PaO$_2$ <8kPa
	Cannot complete sentences	Normal PaCO$_2$ (4.6–6.0 kPa)*
		Silent chest Cyanosis Poor respiratory effort Arrhythmia Exhaustion Altered conscious level Hypotension

6. Suggest a definitive management plan (which includes alerting the appropriate senior)

Management of acute exacerbation of asthma

- Admit all severe and life-threatening cases.
- High-dose **salbutamol nebulisers 2.5–5 mg**
  - High-dose **ipratropium bromide nebulisers 250–500 mcg** can also be used.
- **Oral prednisolone** (40 mg for at least 5 days)
  - 100 mg **IV hydrocortisone** can be used every six hours if oral medications cannot be given.

	• Oxygen, to maintain saturations of 94–98%. • **IV magnesium sulphate** by a specialist, if inadequate response to the above. • **IV aminophylline** by a specialist, if inadequate response to the above. • **Discussion with the intensive care** unit on concerns regarding responses to treatment or life-threatening/near fatal cases.
7. **Briefly discuss the management of the remaining patients**	*Management of delirium tremens* It is important not to jump to conclusions. State to the examiner that for the patient in scenario 2, you would like to take a full history, read through the notes, and complete a thorough examination. • Assessment of severity of symptoms using a scoring system, such as **CIWA**. • Using local guidelines to prescribe background and breakthrough **chlordiazepoxide**. o The frequency and strength of the dose may be titrated against the CIWA score. • Prevention of Wernicke's encephalopathy through the administration of **B12** and **thiamine** (e.g., Pabrinex IV). • Referral to an Alcohol Liaison Nurse. • Referral to dieticians. *Responding to non-medical scenarios* It is important to remain professional at all times whilst at work, which means that you should ensure that your friends and family do not receive attention and treatment that would put the safety and care of others at risk. You must also maintain patient confidentiality as per normal.

Mock Clinical Station 2

You are an FY1 working at a busy hospital on a general medicine firm. You have just put the kettle on in the doctor's mess when you receive the following information:

1. You receive a bleep from a nurse in Ward A who sounds flustered and afraid as she conveys to you that John Jones, a 68-year-old alcoholic, has just vomited up blood and is looking "a little pale". You ask for his obs, which are as follows: sats are 93%, HR is 114, RR is 24, and BP is 88/56. She would like you to review Mr Jones.

2. You receive a bleep from a nurse in Ward B who says that one of her patients, Mr Shirokee, has become very short of breath very quickly. He is not in any pain but is unable to lie flat. He has a history of ischaemic heart disease. His sats are 96% on air, HR is 80, RR is 30, and BP is 116/78.

3. You receive a WhatsApp message from your consultant, who says that they need to urgently access the scans for one of their outpatients on the computer. They are asking you to help them access the images, or could you access the scans yourself and send them across on your phone?

4. Susanne, the HCA on your ward, catches you as you exit and asks if you can sedate Thomas, a 53-year-old man who she suspects has been sneaking alcohol onto the ward. She tells you that he has been shouting abuse at other patients and that they may be distressed.

How would you proceed?

You should use the same structure as in the first clinical example when approaching a station. The key take-home messages for this scenario are as follows:

There is one exception to the A to E rule when it comes to grading the severity of the issue, and that is a catastrophic haemorrhage (the so-called C-ABCDE used by NICE and other recent guidelines). This is because exsanguination poses a rapidly worsening threat to life, with measures that can be put in place to mitigate its effects whilst the definitive cause is sought.

When grading the scenarios, scenario 1 could very well be consistent with a variceal bleed — this would be graded as a "C" for "catastrophic haemorrhage". Scenario 2 would be graded as a "B" initially, scenario 4 would be graded as a "D" and scenario 3 would not be classed as a medical emergency.

5.2.1 *Management of a variceal bleed*

- Activate the **major haemorrhage protocol**.
  - ○ This varies from hospital to hospital but will usually involve the summoning of the crash team, a porter, and the notification of the haematology and blood bank about a patient who will likely require urgent transfusion. Occasionally, blood is made available immediately.
- Protect the airway.
- **Insert two wide-bore cannulae**, preferably in the antecubital fossa.
- Draw off two **Group** and **Save** samples.
- Commence aggressive **fluid resuscitation** whilst awaiting blood products.
- **Urgent discussion with gastroenterology.**
  - ○ Consider urgent endoscopy.
- Consider **pharmacological therapy** (octreotide/vasopressin).
- Consider the **insertion of a tamponade device** (Sengstaken-Blakemore tube).

5.2.2 *Management of acutely decompensated left-sided heart failure*

The patient in scenario 1 has suddenly become short of breath. Whilst there are a number of differentials that must come to mind in acute dyspnoea (PE, pneumothorax, aspiration event, mucous plugging and pulmonary oedema, to name a few), his history of ischaemic heart disease and the inability to lie flat in the absence of chest pain make pulmonary oedema more likely. Note that we initially categorised this acute medical issue as a "B" when, in fact, the underlying aetiology was a "C".

In this scenario, whilst conducting your A to E assessment, you will need to request the appropriate investigations (initially and ABG and a chest X-ray). The management of acute heart failure consists of the following:

- Administer O_2
- **Sit** patient **up**
- Bolus of **diuretics** (e.g., IV furosemide 20–40 mg)
- Consider the use of **nitrates**
- Commence accurate input/output monitoring (may require catherisation)

5.2.3 Information governance

In scenario 3, your consultant is asking you to take photos of scans of patients on your personal device. Pictures and information stored on personal phones are prone to leak and may be accessed by non-healthcare staff and people not responsible for the care of that patient.

For that reason, taking photographs and storing sensitive information about patients on your personal phone should be avoided. You could offer to go down to your consultant after you have dealt with the acute emergencies to help them access the IT systems.

Mock Clinical Station 3

You are an FY1 working a busy District General Hospital on a general medicine firm. You have just finished labelling the bottles of blood from a patient when:

1. You receive a bleep from a nurse in Ward Y asking you to see Gillian, a 24-year-old who started fitting 3 minutes ago. The nurse thinks that Gillian has soiled her bed and is concerned that she is frothing a lot at the mouth. The nurse wonders if you can review the patient and stop the fitting. The patient's sats are unknown, HR is 88, RR is unknown, and BP is 138/80.
2. You are called by your registrar to review a patient who he has just been bleeped about. The patient is Sarthak, a 76-year-old inpatient who has been in hospital for three weeks and whom you know quite well. His HCA is concerned that Sarthak is more confused than usual and has started talking about the "asteroids on the walls, and smurfs in his coffee". She would like you to review him.
3. You walk past an F1 colleague from another firm, who is crouched in the doorway to the stock cupboard, sobbing. She makes eye contact with you as you are walking past her.

How do you proceed?

Once again, apply the A to E rule to categorise these vignettes based on their severity.

It would be an easy (yet unforgivable) mistake to categorise scenario 1 as a "D". The patient is fitting and should be presumed to have lost his airway until you have managed to assess him. **This is a medical emergency** and usually warrants putting out a medical emergency or peri-arrest call.

Scenario 2 is an elderly patient with new onset confusion. This should be categorised as a "D". Note that there are a number of different causes of sudden onset confusion, and one of your differentials should include a stroke (particularly if the patient had a history of strokes or was an arteriopath). Since the management of strokes is time-critical, it might be sensible to inform a colleague and see if they could provide help whilst you go to the patient in scenario 1.

Scenario 3 is not a medical emergency but should still be dealt with sensitivity and compassion.

5.2.4 *Management of a fitting patient*

The most important aspect of the management of this patient is to secure an airway. If you have any concerns, and the patient is requiring airway support in the form of an oropharyngeal or nasopharyngeal airway, you need to ensure that anaesthetics are on hand.

The management of the fitting patient is as follows:

- Secure the **airway**.
- Administer 15L of high-flow **oxygen** and continue to monitor saturations.
- Secure **IV access**:
  - Ideally 2x large-bore cannula.
  - Draw off bloods and gas.
- Terminate the seizure:
  - First line: **IV lorazepam 4 mg** or PR diazepam 10 mg.
  - Second line: **IV lorazepam 4 mg** after 10 minutes.
  - Third line: **phenytoin infusion** (15–18 mg/kg).
- Look for any **underlying cause and reverse**:
  - ECG
  - Blood glucose
  - Electrolytes (sodium, potassium, magnesium, calcium)

  ○ CT head
  ○ (Later) EEG

Note that if the second dose of lorazepam has failed to terminate the seizure, then phenytoin will need to be given by a senior clinician or an anaesthetist, with the next management step being general anaesthesia. It is worth committing the doses of lorazepam and diazepam to memory, although note that weight-based doses will be used in children. If in doubt, always check the BNF.

If a scenario arises in your interview about a fitting patient, you also need to be prepared to answer questions about the different causes of seizures. It is useful to place these causes into categories to help you remember them. There are a number of different ways of categorising the causes and the one provided below is one of many, and this list is non-exhaustive:

- Neurological

  ○ Epilepsy
  ○ Space occupying lesion
  ○ Meningitis/encephalitis
  ○ Stroke

- Cardiac/Respiratory

  ○ Any cardiac or respiratory disorder causing secondary anoxic seizures
  ○ Arrythmias

- Metabolic

  ○ Hyper/hypoglycaemia
  ○ Abnormalities of:

    ▪ Sodium
    ▪ Potassium
    ▪ Magnesium
    ▪ Calcium
    ▪ Phosphate

  ○ Toxins, e.g.,
    ▪ Uraemia
    ▪ ETOH
    ▪ Drugs, including: cocaine and amphetamines
    ▪ Toxin withdrawal

  ○ Malignant hypertension

Once a cause has been identified, efforts should be made to reverse the underlying cause.

5.2.5 Management of acute delirium

The management of a delirious patient relies firstly on conducting a comprehensive A to E assessment. Following this, a full **neurological assessment** should be performed, including examination of the cranial nerves, and nerves of the limbs. A "delirium screen" is often performed in these situations. The management of a delirious patient can therefore be summarised as follows:

- Perform an A to E assessment.
- Conduct neurological examination.
- "Delirium screen"
  - ECG
  - Blood glucose
  - Urine dip
  - Consider Chest X-ray if there is a suspicion of
  - Consider CT head (particularly if there is concern about an intracranial event)
  - Bloods
    - FBC
    - U&Es
    - Bone profile
    - Magnesium
    - B12, folate, iron studies
    - Vitamin D
    - Thyroid function tests
    - Liver function tests

Some patients demonstrate hyperactive delirium and may become aggressive or violent towards other patients or other members of staff. These patients should be risk assessed and following discussion with the patient's family and at the discretion of the consultant responsible for their care, a DoLS (Deprivation of Liberty Safeguarding) may have to be put in place to allow further treatment.

Mock Clinical Station 3

You are an FY1 working in a busy District General Hospital in a general medicine firm. You have had probably the worst fish and chips meal from the hospital canteen, and it cost you £8.30. You paid extra for a drink. You're irritated, when:

1. You are bleeped about a 17-year-old patient, Michelle, who was previously admitted with an asthma attack and is now vomiting and complaining of severe abdominal pain. Observations are as follows: her HR is 104, BP is 130/80, sats 100% on room air, and RR is 44. The nurse is concerned about how laboured the patient's breaths are.
2. You receive a bleep from a nurse in the Pixie ward asking you to see Isabella, a 67-year-old who started feeling "funniness in the chest" 20 minutes ago. The nurse says it is her first day and doesn't know what to do.
3. Your registrar asks you to look over his job application, which is due in a few hours.

How do you proceed?

Note: some parameters may be available to the interviewee should they request them; these are available in the feedback below.

Using the A to E strategy to categorise these patients, scenario 1 is peculiar since it is a combination of abdominal pain and severe tachypnoea in a patient with a background of asthma, but it would be safer to categorise it as a "B" — a respiratory rate of 40 and the nurse commenting about the intensity of the breathing should prompt an urgent review.

There is very little information in the vignette in scenario 2, but any patient with chest pain should have an ECG to rule out ischaemia, infarction or arrhythmias. This would come under a "C", and although this scenario is below the first in terms of priority, it would be sensible to ask for an ECG in the first instance. Once again, informing your SHO that there are multiple sick patients that need your attention is a good idea, since they may be able to help you.

The third scenario is clearly not a medical emergency.

For the first scenario, you should approach it once again using your A to E approach. Assuming her airway is patent, you should then proceed to assessing patient "B" (breathing). For this scenario, the interviewers would likely provide you with the following additional information:

Assessment Component	Findings
Obs	Saturations 100% on 6L Respiratory rate 44
Peripheral Assessment	Patient tachypnoeic Deep, laboured breathing Unable to complete sentences
Central Assessment	Trachea central and non-deviated Equal and symmetrical chest rise Chest clear Nil added breath sounds

From the information above, the patient is clearly in respiratory distress, but the normal saturations and the absence of signs on clinical examination suggest that the underlying cause is not respiratory.

At this stage, you should complete your assessment of patient "B" and:

- Request for a chest X-ray
- Perform an ABG if

    i) there is evidence of desaturation or
    ii) the patient is in respiratory distress

Your ABG (on 6L) therefore demonstrates the following results:

pH	7.2
pCO_2	2.1 kPa
pO_2	16.8 kPa
BE	−8.0 mEq/L
HCO_3	14 mmol/L
sO_2	99.6%

Lactate	0.8 mmol/L
Glucose	32.3 mmol/L

Note that you should be aware of the normal values for blood gas measurement. For completeness, however, the normal ranges are listed below.

pH	7.35–7.45
pCO_2	4.6–6.4 kPa
pO_2	11.0–14.4 kPa
BE	–2–2 mEq/L
HCO_3	22–26 mmol/L
sO_2	94–98%
Lactate	0.5–2.2 mmol/L
Glucose	3.6–5.3 mmol/L

This blood gas shows a profound **metabolic acidosis**. The glucose is very high, and in a young patient presenting with tachypnoea and abdominal pain, you should be thinking about **diabetic ketoacidosis** as the first presentation of type 1 diabetes.

5.2.6 *Management of diabetic ketoacidosis*

- Commence **fixed rate insulin infusion**
  - 50 units of actrapid in 50 mls of normal saline to be run at 0.1 mls/ kg/hour.
- **Fluid resuscitation**
  - If systolic BP is under 90, give 500 ml of fluid bolus.
  - Fluid resuscitation is aggressive, consisting of
    - 1L in the first hour
    - Two bags of 1L to run over two hours each
    - Two further bags of 1L to run over four hours each

- ○ When BMs are above 14 mmol/L, use normal saline as fluid.
- ○ When BMs are below 14 mmol/L, use 5% dextrose as fluid.

- **Monitor BMs and ketones** regularly to ensure improvement:
  - ○ At least hourly initially
  - ○ Aim for a reduction in BM of 3 mmol/L/hour
  - ○ Aim for a ketone reduction of 0.5 mmol/L/hour

- **Monitor potassium** carefully:
  - ○ Consider adding 20 mmol of potassium chloride from the second bag of fluids onwards
  - ○ Monitor at 60 minutes, two hours and then every two hours, thereafter

- **Continue blood glucose and ketone** monitoring until ketones <0.3 mmol/L and the pH is above 7.3, **and the** patient is able to **eat and drink.**

The patient should be referred to an endocrinologist or diabetic specialist nurse whilst on the infusion and should be commenced on subcutaneous insulin therapy before the fixed rate insulin infusion is stopped. Weaning and stopping of insulin infusions should be performed by a senior.

5.2.7 *Management of acute myocardial infarction*

The assessment and management of DKA will likely take up most of the interview time, but you should also be briefly aware of the management of myocardial infarction. Acute cardiac-sounding chest pain is usually labelled as one of the following:

i. ST-segment elevation myocardial infarction (STEMI)
ii. Non-ST-segment elevation myocardial infarction (NSTEMI)
iii. Unstable angina
iv. Stable angina

The classification of these is based on the presence of (a) whether the pain occurs at rest, (b) ECG changes, and (c) troponin changes.

Diagnosis	Chest pain	Common ECG changes*	Troponin
STEMI	Cardiac sounding A rest	ST-segment elevation Anterior lead ST depression (possible posterior STEMI)	Elevated
NSTEMI	Cardiac sounding A rest	ST-segment depression T wave inversion	Elevated
Unstable angina	Cardiac sounding A rest	Usually none	Not elevated
Stable angina	Cardiac sounding Exertional Relieved by rest	Usually none	

Note that these are the common ECG changes, and there are numerous other changes that may be noted.

The first step is to diagnose appropriately. As part of your A to E approach, you will request an ECG. If there is evidence of ST-elevation, then the condition should be treated as STEMI (ST-elevation myocardial infarction) and be managed as follows:

- Oxygen, if hypoxic.
- Send at least two troponins separated by at least four hours (depending on troponin sensitivity used by your Trust).
- Discuss the patient with your nearest HACU (hyper-acute cardiac unit) for consideration of urgent PCI (percutaneous coronary intervention) or thrombolysis.
- Commence on the following medications:
  - Load with aspirin 300 mg
  - Load with clopidogrel 300 mg or ticagrelor 180 mg
  - Fondaparinux 2.5 mg (to be continued for 3–5 days)
  - GTN spray PRN for chest pain
    - This can be converted to a GTN infusion titrated to achieve a resolution of chest pain

- ○ Morphine 10 mg
- ○ Metoclopramide 10 mg

You should also commence the following long-term medications, as long as there are no contraindications:

- Beta blockers, e.g., bisoprolol
- High dose statins, e.g., atorvastatin
- ACE inhibitors, e.g., ramipril

The management of an NSTEMI is similar to the above.

5.3 Academic Interview Stations

Mock Academic Station 1[1]

BACKGROUND

Short-term survival benefits of endovascular aneurysm repair (EVAR) versus open repair of intact abdominal aortic aneurysms have been shown in randomised trials. However, this early survival benefit is lost after a few years. We investigated whether EVAR had a long-term survival benefit compared with open repair.

METHODS

We used data from the EVAR randomised controlled trial (EVAR trial 1), which enrolled 1,252 patients from 37 centres in the UK between 1 September 1999 and 31 August 2004. Patients had to be aged 60 years or older, have aneurysms that were at least 5.5 cm in diameter, and be deemed suitable and fit for either EVAR or open repair. Eligible patients were randomly assigned (1:1) using computer-generated sequences of randomly permuted blocks stratified by the centre to receive either EVAR (n = 626) or open repair (n = 626). Patients and treating clinicians were aware of group assignments; no masking was used. The primary analysis compared total and aneurysm-related deaths in groups until mid-2015 in the intention-to-treat population. This trial is registered at ISRCTN (ISRCTN55703451).

FINDINGS

Of the 1,252 patients recruited, 25 (four for mortality outcome) were lost over follow-ups by 30 June 2015. Over a mean of 12.7 years (SD 1.5; maximum 15.8 years) of follow-ups, we recorded 9.3 deaths per

100 person-years in the EVAR group and 8.9 deaths per 100 person-years in the open-repair group (adjusted hazard ratio [HR] 1.11, 95% CI 0.97 to 1.27, p = 0.14). At 0–6 months after randomisation, patients in the EVAR group had a lower mortality (adjusted HR 0.61, 95% CI 0·37 to 1.02 for total mortality; and 0.47, 0.23 to 0.93 for aneurysm-related mortality, p = 0·031). However, beyond eight years of follow-ups, open-repair had a significantly lower mortality (adjusted HR 1,25, 95% CI 1,00 to 1,56, p = 0.048 for total mortality; and 5.82, 1.64 to 20.65, p = 0.0064 for aneurysm-related mortality). The increased aneurysm-related mortality in the EVAR group after eight years was mainly attributable to secondary aneurysm sac rupture (13 deaths [7%] in EVAR versus two [1%] in open repair), with increased cancer mortality also observed in the EVAR group.

INTERPRETATION

EVAR has an early survival benefit but an inferior late survival rate as compared with open repair, which needs to be addressed by lifelong surveillance of EVAR and re-intervention, if necessary.

FUNDING

UK National Institute for Health Research, Camelia Botnar Arterial Research Foundation.

Please summarise this study and critically appraise it.

| 1. Summary of the study | • **Design:** This is a multi-centre randomised controlled trial.
 • **Population:** 1,252 patients who were >60 years old, with ≥5.5 cm aneurysms and were fit for surgery.
 • **Intervention:** EVAR
 • **Control:** Open Repair
 • **Outcome(s):** total and aneurysm related deaths.
 • **Summary of findings:** EVAR has an early survival benefit, but this is not the case in the long term. |

2. Internal validity	**Study design:**
	• This is a multi-centre randomised controlled trial, which is high on the hierarchy of evidence and reduces selection bias.
	Population:
	• Large sample size, n = 1,252; it would be important to check the power calculation in the full text.
	• Inclusion/exclusion criteria: the definition of severe aortic stenosis is clearly defined, which allows for reproducibility. It would be important to check how the authors defined "asymptomatic" (was this patient reported or criteria formed?). Given that aortic stenosis occurs in older patients, it would be important to check the baseline demographics of both groups for comorbidities, which could affect the results.
	Intervention:
	• No blinding was used but this is difficult in surgery as patients can tell from the scars which operation they have undergone.
	• This is offset by the use of objective primary endpoints (death).
	Outcomes:
	• The primary outcome was objective — deaths related to aneurysm and total deaths.
	• A follow-up time of 12.7 years, which is long but in vascular patients this may be insufficient
	• No patient-reported or functional outcomes are described in the abstract; it would be important to check the full-text for any patient-reported symptomatic improvements post-surgery.
	Statistics:
	• An intention-to-treat analysis was used, which means that all subjects randomised to the

	treatment arms were included in the final analyses with the advantage of mirroring "real-life" practice.
3. External validity	• The study was multi-centre, which increases its generalisability. • The study reporting would benefit from a cost-effectiveness analysis or a number needed to treat calculation with respect to early surgery, preventing deaths. • It would also be good to know the demographics of the two groups, which were randomised, as this would allow us to investigate whether the findings are generalisable, and whether any confounders may have accounted for the results. • We also do not know the proportion of these who were emergency operations or elective, which would be useful when considering the application of EVAR.
4. Ethics	• I would like to check the paper to ensure consent was obtained from all the participants. • I would also like to check if the trial investigators had set parameters under which they would terminate the trial, i.e., if they noticed a significant difference between the groups, they would terminate the trial as one group would be benefiting more than the other.

Mock Academic Station 2[2]

BACKGROUND

For women with oestrogen receptor (ER)-positive early breast cancer, treatment with tamoxifen for five years substantially reduces the breast cancer mortality rate throughout the first 15 years after diagnosis. We aimed to assess the effects of continuing tamoxifen for ten years instead of five years.

Mock Academic Station 2[2]

METHODS

In the worldwide Adjuvant Tamoxifen: Longer Against Shorter (ATLAS) trial, 12,894 women with early breast cancer who had completed five years of treatment with tamoxifen were randomly selected to continue with tamoxifen up to ten years or stop at the 5-year (open control) mark. The allocation (1:1) was done by a central computer, using minimisation. After entry (between 1996 and 2005), yearly follow-up forms recorded any recurrences, second cancer, hospital admissions, or death. We report effects on breast cancer outcomes among the 6,846 women with ER-positive disease and side effects among all women (with positive, negative, or unknown ER status). Long-term follow-up still continues. This study is registered, number ISRCTN19652633.

FINDINGS

Among women with ER-positive disease, allocation to continue tamoxifen reduced the risk of breast cancer recurrence (617 recurrences in 3,428 women allocated to continue versus 711 in 3,418 controls, p = 0.002), reduced breast cancer mortality (331 deaths versus 397 deaths, p = 0.01), and reduced overall mortality (639 deaths versus 722 deaths, p = 0.01). The reductions in adverse breast cancer outcomes appeared to be less extreme before year 10 (recurrence rate ratio [RR] 0.90 [95% CI 0.79 to 1.02] during years 5–9 and 0.75 [0.62 to 0.90] in later years; breast cancer mortality RR 0.97 [0.79 to 1.18] during years 5–9 and 0.71 [0.58 to 0.88] in later years). The cumulative risk of recurrence during years 5–14 was 21.4% for women allocated to continue versus 25.1% for controls; breast cancer mortality during years 5–14 was 12.2% for women allocated to continue versus 15.0% for controls (absolute mortality reduction 2.8%). Treatment allocation seemed to have no effect on breast cancer outcome among 1,248 women with ER-negative disease, and an intermediate effect among 4,800 women with an unknown ER status. Among all 12,894 women, mortality without recurrence from causes other than breast cancer was only slightly affected (688 deaths without recurrence in 6,454 women allocated to continue versus 679 deaths in the 6,440 controls; RR 0.99 [0.89 to 1.10]; p = 0.78). For the incidence (hospitalisation or death) rates of specific diseases, RRs were as follows: pulmonary embolus 1.87 (95% CI 1.13 to 3.07, p = 0·01 [including 0.2% mortality in both treatment groups]), stroke 1.06 (0.83 to 1.36), ischaemic heart

Mock Academic Station 2[2]

disease 0.75 (0.60 to 0.95, p = 0.02), and endometrial cancer 1.74 (1.30 to 2.34, p = 0·0002). The cumulative risk of endometrial cancer during years 5–14 was 3.1% (mortality 0.4%) for women allocated to continue versus 1.6% (mortality 0.2%) for the controls (absolute mortality increase 0.2%).

INTERPRETATION

For women with ER-positive disease, continuing tamoxifen for ten years rather than stopping at five years produce a further reduction in recurrence and mortality, particularly after year 10. These results, taken together with results from previous trials of five years of tamoxifen treatment versus none, suggest that ten years of tamoxifen treatment can approximately halve breast cancer mortality during the second decade after diagnosis.

FUNDING

Cancer Research UK, UK Medical Research Council, AstraZeneca UK, US Army, EU-Biomed.

The examiner should ask the questions outlined below in the suggested approach.

Summary of the Study	<ul><li>Design: Randomised controlled trial.</li><li>P: 12,894 women with early breast cancer who had completed five years of treatment with tamoxifen.</li><li>I: continue tamoxifen up to ten years of treatment.</li><li>C: stop tamoxifen treatment at five years (open control).</li><li>O: breast cancer outcome, including recurrence, second cancer, hospital admission, or death, and side effects of treatment.</li></ul> Summarise main findings: Overall, the study results showed that continuing tamoxifen to ten years versus stopping at five years significantly reduced cancer recurrence and the mortality rate.

What are Some Strengths of This Study?	Some points could include: • RCT with long-term follow-up: high on the hierarchy of evidence. • Large sample size. • Long follow-up time (ten years) and an ongoing study. • External Validity: multi-centre, widely available study drug, safety risks were assessed along with clinical efficacy. Negatives: open control (i.e., no blinding)
What Do You Think About the Outcomes?	The study outcomes are good because they consider clinical efficacy (recurrence, death, hospital admissions) as well as safety (e.g., PE, endometrial cancer, cardiovascular disease, etc.). Other outcomes they could have included: patient-reported outcomes (quality of life taking tamoxifen, minor side effects).
How Would You Explain These Results to a Patient?	Women with early stage breast cancer (i.e., breast cancer which has not spread elsewhere), who took the study drug (tamoxifen) for ten years, had lower rates of their cancer returning, and of death, than women who only took the drug for five years.
Should We Change Our Practice Based on This Study?	I would like to have further information before making a decision — a large meta-analysis and systematic review being the highest quality evidence on the hierarchy of evidence-based medicine. Overall, this is a large, well-designed study with a relatively long follow-up time, so it probably should inform clinical practice.

Mock Academic Station 3[3]

BACKGROUND

In randomised trials, fecal occult blood testing reduces mortality from colorectal cancer. However, the duration of the benefit is unknown, as are the effects specific to age and sex.

METHODS

In the Minnesota Colon Cancer Control Study, 46,551 participants, 50 to 80 years of age, were randomly assigned to usual care (control) or to annual or biennial screening with fecal occult blood testing. The screening was performed from 1976 through 1982 and from 1986 through 1992. We used the National Death Index to obtain updated information on the vital status of participants and to determine the causes of death through 2008.

RESULTS

Through 30 years of follow-up, 33,020 participants (70.9%) died. A total of 732 deaths were attributed to colorectal cancer: 200 of the 11,072 deaths (1.8%) in the annual screening group, 237 of the 11,004 deaths (2.2%) in the biennial screening group, and 295 of the 10,944 deaths (2.7%) in the control group. Screening reduced colorectal cancer mortality (relative risk with annual screening, 0.68; 95% confidence interval [CI], 0.56 to 0.82; relative risk with biennial screening, 0.78; 95% CI, 0.65 to 0.93) through 30 years of follow-ups. No reduction was observed in all-cause mortality (relative risk with annual screening, 1.00; 95% CI, 0.99 to 1.01; relative risk with biennial screening, 0.99; 95% CI, 0.98 to 1.01). The reduction in colorectal cancer mortality was larger for men than for women in the biennial-screening group ($P = 0.04$ for interaction).

CONCLUSIONS

The effect of screening with fecal occult blood testing on colorectal cancer mortality persists after 30 years but does not influence all-cause mortality. The sustained reduction in colorectal cancer mortality supports the effect of polypectomy. (Funded by the Veterans Affairs Merit Review Award Program and others.)

The examiner should ask the questions outlined below in the suggested approach.

Summary of the Study	• Design: • **P:** 46,551 participants, 50 to 80 years of age. • **I:** annual or biennial screening with faecal occult-blood testing. • **C:** usual care. • **O:** mortality (colorectal cancer mortality and all-cause mortality). Overall, the study found that screening with faecal occult-blood testing reduced colorectal cancer mortality after 30 years but did not influence all-cause mortality.
What are Some Strengths and Weaknesses of This Study Design?	The pros of this study design (RCT) include: • Gold standard for studying treatment effects. • Random allocation reduces selection bias and equally distributes confounding factors between treatment arms. • It is prospective, i.e., allows one to conclude causation between intervention and outcome. • There is a large number of participants (likely to be well powered, but this should be checked in the full paper. • There is a long follow-up time of 30 years. The cons of this study design include: • Difficult to set up and maintain. • They are time-consuming and expensive. • There are ethical problems in giving different treatments to the groups.
What are the Ethical Implications of This Study?	• The main ethical implication of this study design is centred around the principle of beneficence/non-maleficence. • Participants who received screening with fecal occult blood testing had significantly lower rates of colorectal cancer-specific mortality

	than those who were not screened. Hence it could be argued that it was not ethical to randomise people NOT to have a potentially life-saving intervention.
	• However, the opposing argument would be that the study IS ethical because fecal occult blood testing at the time was not established practice; hence this study needed to be conducted to prove that screening was worthwhile for patients to benefit on a population scale.
	• A good compromise (which would most likely happen in modern research practice) would be to conduct interim analyses, such that if a significant benefit was detected early on, all participants (including the control group) could receive the beneficial intervention.
How Would You Explain These Results to a Patient?	Women with early-stage breast cancer (i.e., breast cancer which has not spread elsewhere), who took the study drug (tamoxifen) for ten years, had lower rates of the cancer returning, and of death, than women who only took the drug for five years.
Are the Results Statistically Significant?	The significant results in this study included: • Significant reduction in colorectal cancer mortality: the risk ratios were less than 1 and the confidence intervals for annual and biennial screening **did not cross 1, making this result significant**. • The reduction in colorectal cancer mortality was significantly larger for men than for women in the biennial-screening group; p was **<0.05 ($p = 0.04$), making this result significant**.

However, there was no significant reduction in all-cause mortality: the relative risk with annual screening was 0.99 to 1, and the confidence interval **crossed 1** for both the annual and biennial screening, **making this result non-significant**.

Mock Academic Station 4[4]

BACKGROUND

Symptomatic relief is the primary goal of percutaneous coronary intervention (PCI) in stable angina and is commonly observed clinically. However, there is no evidence from blinded, placebo-controlled randomised trials to show its efficacy.

METHODS

ORBITA is a blinded, multi-centre randomised trial of PCI versus a placebo procedure for angina relief done at five study sites in the UK. We enrolled patients with severe (≥70%) single-vessel stenoses. After enrolment, patients received six weeks of medication optimisation. Patients then had pre-randomisation assessments with cardiopulmonary exercise testing, symptom questionnaires, and dobutamine stress echocardiography. Patients were randomised 1:1 to undergo PCI or a placebo procedure by use of an automated online randomisation tool. After six weeks of follow-up, the assessments done before randomisation were repeated at the final assessment. The primary endpoint was the difference in exercise time increment between groups. All analyses were based on the intention-to-treat principle, and the study population contained all participants who underwent randomisation. This study is registered with ClinicalTrials.gov, number NCT02062593.

FINDINGS

ORBITA enrolled 230 patients with ischaemic symptoms. After the medication optimisation phase and between 6 Jan 2014 and 11 Aug 2017, 200 patients underwent randomisation, with 105 patients assigned PCI and 95 assigned the placebo procedure. Lesions had mean area stenosis of 84.4% (SD 10.2), a fractional flow reserve of

0.69 (0.16), and an instantaneous wave-free ratio of 0.76 (0.22). There was no significant difference in the primary endpoint of exercise time increment between the groups (PCI minus placebo 16.6 s, 95% CI −8.9 to 42.0, p = 0.200). There were no deaths. Serious adverse events included four pressure-wire related complications in the placebo group, which required PCI, and five major bleeding events, including two in the PCI group and three in the placebo group.

INTERPRETATION

In patients with medically treated angina and severe coronary stenosis, PCI did not increase exercise time by more than the effect of a placebo procedure. The efficacy of invasive procedures can be assessed with a placebo control, as is standard for pharmacotherapy.

FUNDING

NIHR Imperial Biomedical Research Centre, Foundation for Circulatory Health, Imperial College Healthcare Charity, Philips Volcano, NIHR Barts Biomedical Research Centre.

The examiner should ask the questions outlined below in the suggested approach.

Summarise This Study in Lay Terms	This study found that in people with angina with one severely blocked artery supplying the heart, there was no difference between stenting the artery versus using only medicines in terms of "exercise time" (time taken for people to walk without stopping due to chest pain).
What are Some Strengths and Weaknesses of This Study?	The strengths of study design include: • Gold standard for studying treatment effects. • Random allocation reduces selection bias and equally distributes confounding factors between treatment arms. • Prospective: allows one to conclude causation between intervention and outcome.

- The study was blinded, to reduce observation/detection bias.
- The outcomes were designed *a priori* (the study has a trials number).
- An intention-to-treat principle was used in the statistical analysis.

The weaknesses of this study design include:

- Difficult to maintain, time-consuming and expensive.
- May be sponsored by for-profit companies, i.e., *Philips Volcano*, in this case.
- The data is limited to participants from the UK.
- The follow up time is relatively short (six weeks).
- Mortality was not assessed (the main outcome was exercise time increment).
- There are ethical problems in giving different treatments to the groups.

What is the Intention to Treat Principle? What is the Strength of Using This Method?	• The intention to treat principle stipulates that all subjects randomised in the study are included in the analyses as members of the groups they were allocated, regardless of whether they completed the study. This means that patients who are randomised but then subsequently drop out or switch groups are still included in the analyses. • The advantage of this method is that it "mirrors" real-life practice. For example, some participants may drop out of a study due to the side effects of the study drug. Dropping out early might mean that the study drug appears less effective because it was taken for a shorter period of time, but it gives a more holistic view. There is no point using a very effective study drug that few would take due to side effects!

Should We Change Our Practice Based on This Paper?	• When answering this question, I would look at the strength and generalisability of the evidence. This is a well-designed randomised-controlled, blinded trial with results that suggest no improvement in exercise tolerance with PCI versus best medical therapy in the first six weeks. • However, the data was limited to a relatively small sample (200) of UK patients. Furthermore, mortality and cardiovascular events were not included outcomes. It would therefore be difficult to justify withholding PCI to symptomatic patients on the basis of this evidence without knowing the long-term effects. • Overall, no, PCI should not be withheld on the basis of this evidence, but the study should encourage another, longer and similarly well-designed trial looking at long-term outcomes.
Patients in This Study Allocated to the Control Group Underwent a "placebo procedure", i.e., an invasive procedure without therapeutic intervention, otherwise known as a "sham control". What are the Ethical Implications of This?	This study raises important ethical questions related to the four principles of medical ethics. • Non-maleficence: 　○ The study withheld a gold standard, potentially beneficial treatment (PCI) from participants. Arterial catheterisation is not a benign procedure, and patients in the control group were put at risk of pressure-wire related complications and major bleeding events. • Beneficence: 　○ Proponents of the study could argue that although the study put patients at risk in the placebo group, there was a "net" good effect. 　○ Patients who underwent the placebo had the opportunity to undergo PCI at the end of the trial when it became unblinded (only a 6-week wait, and most likely faster than current NHS waiting lists!)

> - Also, regardless of the intervention, all patients benefitted from a thorough assessment of their symptoms and medicines optimisation.
> - Autonomy:
>   - Patients have the right to take part in trials if they give informed consent.
>   - One could argue whether patients who hadn't had PCI before they understood the risks of this invasive procedure and the potential serious adverse effects.
> - Justice/utilitarianism:
>   - Putting patients at the risk of invasive procedures is justified if the results could potentially improve clinical practice on a population scale.

5.4 References

1. Patel R, Sweeting MJ, Powell JT, Greenhalgh RM. (2016) EVAR trial investigators. Endovascular versus open repair of abdominal aortic aneurysm in 15-years' follow-up of the UK endovascular aneurysm repair trial 1 (EVAR trial 1): A randomised controlled trial. *Lancet* **388**(10058): 2366–74. doi:10.1016/S0140-6736(16)31135-7.
2. Davies C, Pan H, Godwin J, *et al.* (2013) Long-term effects of continuing adjuvant tamoxifen to 10 years versus stopping at 5 years after diagnosis of oestrogen receptor-positive breast cancer: ATLAS, a randomised trial. *Lancet* **381**(9869): 805–16.
3. Shaukat A, Mongin SJ, Geisser MS, *et al.* (2013) Long-term mortality after screening for colorectal cancer. (2013). *N Engl J Med* **369**(12): 1106–14. doi: 10.1056/NEJMoa1300720.
4. Al-Lamee R, Thompson D, Dehbi H, *et al.* (2018) Percutaneous coronary intervention in stable angina (ORBITA): A double-blind, randomised controlled trial. *Lancet* **391**(10115): 31–40.

Printed in Great Britain
by Amazon

30635733R00075